Free Gift

with

PURCHASE

Jean Godfrey-June

my improbable career in magazines and makeup

Free Gift with PURCHASE

harmony books / new york

Published in the United States by Harmony Books, an imprint of the Crown Publishing Group, a division of Random House, Inc., New York.
www.crownpublishing.com

Harmony Books is a registered trademark and the Harmony Books colophon is a trademark of Random House, Inc.

Library of Congress Cataloging-in-Publication Data

Godfrey-June, Jean, 1964–
Free gift with purchase : my improbable career in magazines and makeup / Jean Godfrey-June.
p. cm.
1. Godfrey-June, Jean, 1964– 2. Image consultants—United States—Biography. 3. Fashion writers—United States—Biography. 4. Beauty, Personal—United States. I. Title.
TT505.G63A3 2006
646.7'042'092—dc22
2005023522

ISBN-13: 978-0-307-23748-4
ISBN-10: 0-307-23748-6

Printed in the United States of America

DESIGN BY ELINA D. NUDELMAN

10 9 8 7 6 5 4 3 2 1

First Edition

To my teachers

“Beauty?
I would love her with all my heart,
if only she were a goddess and immortal.”

—Charles Baudelaire

Acknowledgments

Thank you: Gary June, India June, Wiley June, Adam Smith, Hilton Als, Kim France, Lydia Wills, Mayer Rus, Jennifer Scruby, Shaye Areheart, Kimberly Kanner Meisner, Liz Flahive, Cristina Mueller, and Dawn Spinner.

Contents

Free Gift

with

PURCHASE

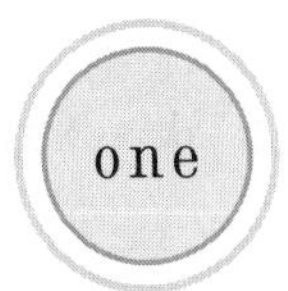

I Know You Are, but What Am I?

You know all the studies, how beautiful people make more money, do better in school, etc., etc., than everyone else? I think when you look at a truly beautiful person, you think, We're still the same species, no? If humanity shares 95 percent of its DNA with a fruit fly, how much must I be sharing with this gorgeous person here? You want to think you're a little like them.

I am not, never was, and never will be a beautiful woman. I'm perfectly lovely, and I feel confident in my powers to fulfill whatever sexual and/or romantic aspirations I might have. But turn-heads-take-breath-away beautiful, no.

Like if I were the next person after you to go out with your ex-boyfriend, you'd see me at a party and think, *Oh, OK*. Whereas if I looked like Kate Moss or Sophia Loren, you might freak out a little.

I used to think I was ugly. I guess everyone does: Models are always going on about how hideous they thought they were and everyone teased them and then suddenly they found themselves in St. Barts getting $10,000 a day to have their picture taken. At first, it wasn't even about "ugly" per se: I was concerned only that people would mistake me for a boy. Gender issues.

My mother likes short hair. She and *her* mother, Grandma Helen (generally a more pro-glamour operative, but she toed the line on short hair), were at their happiest during the Dorothy Hamill period. "Doesn't she look *nice*?" was the refrain of the day, wherever we went, wherever the shiny ducktails would bob no-nonsensely past. My hair at the time was very early Kurt Cobain (minus the bleach) and a source of great tension among us. All I cared was that it was long, so people would understand that I was a girl.

My mother is anti-glamour through and through: Physical appearances mean nothing to her, despite the fact that she herself is stunningly attractive and, indeed, has plenty of glamour to throw around; she steadfastly refuses to acknowledge it. I spent my childhood wading through mud pits and setting up tents in the middle of blizzards, eating wheat bread and wearing battered pairs of Toughskins on what seemed like one endless hiking expedition.

Pre the Dorothy Hamill era, when I was too small to have much influence on my hairstyle, she kept my hair in a pixie (so cute, so sprightly, right?); everyone thought I was a boy. "So how old are your boys?" I remember some jovial park ranger asking my parents, then bending down with a lollipop or something: "Well, hello there, mister!"

I stared at him coldly until my little sister finally broke down and took a lollipop.

On a school trip to Angel Island when I was six, I had to be "rescued" from the shallows of San Francisco Bay when I refused to respond to the teachers' aides calling me in from the shore: "Little boy, little boy . . ."

I don't see a little boy, do you? was the expression I made that they were too far away to see. I shrugged and ran my hands through the thigh-deep water and concentrated on other things, so as not to hear the shrill, urgent warnings. I thought about shells or sea urchins or something; some irritated mother or aide or teacher eventually came roaring out, perhaps splattering her smock dress with seawater, further irritated to find me unalarmed, nonchalant, defiant.

I bit a mustachioed hairdresser badly on one occasion as he bent over me in the big beige chair by the shampoo sink one day. The shop was one of those mini-mall hair salons that smell violently of wet, snipped hair and mysterious chemicals. I watched the bits of hair—featherish and a lighter brown than I associated with the hair on my head—fall like large itchy tears onto the tarpish plastic "gown" Velcroed around my neck; the shears clipped in their grinding, icy metallic fashion. A scuffle ensued; somehow I managed to draw blood.

A second hairdresser was sent out to finish the job. He cut it even shorter, in big dramatic swaths that sailed to the floor—a cream-colored linoleum embossed with rivulets of gold sparkles that ran through it like ore—in clumps. "See, you look so pretty now," the second hairdresser said in a tone that might have reflected vengeance or pity.

That night I suggested that my little sister give her doll a haircut. (We had new dolls: Hers had brown hair, I had grabbed for the blond.) It took some convincing. "No!" she screamed. I got the scissors, the red-handled for-right-handers-only ones, so she could do it herself.

"She'll look really pretty," I assured her. "Maybe I'll cut my doll's hair when you're through."

I went to the other room and got the green-handled scissors

as a show of good faith. Her doll got a very chic Louise Brooks bob; mine, as you can probably imagine, decided in the end to keep hers long.

I never thought about the fact that I felt ugly until one day in the second grade, when I woke up with a bloody nose that wouldn't stop; the ordeal involved a trip to the hospital, but I was fine. I showed up to school a little late, my nose still encrusted with dried blood but fine. "I'm not going to play with you today," said Julia Ann, the richest little girl in my class, a girl so rich she wore a floor-length dress with her long blond, doll-like hair every day, possessed a dollhouse that was an exact copy of her own glorious mansion, and had ridden in a helicopter with Richard Nixon himself. (I know I'm stacking the deck, but I have to add one more thing: On Halloween, little Julia Ann wanted to be a southern belle, so her parents dressed her in an authentic—meaning actual antique—southern belle costume in precisely her second-grade size, right down to the miniature antique southern belle shoes that fit and the miniature antique southern belle parasol by her side.) "I'm not going to play with you today," said Julia Ann, looking at my nose uncomfortably. "You're ugly."

Even after the nose had healed, the fact was still there: Beyond the boy hair, I had freckles. And the attendant pale, blotchy skin. I lived in California, where everyone was tawny and smooth and honey colored and fringed with pool-bleached, longer-than-a-pixie hair.

I'd like to say I've moved past these obsessions, but the truth, as your therapist will tell you, is that people rarely make it past the world of childhood. To this day, my hair is long, long, or longer. Someday (God willing, etc.) I'll grow into one of those disconcerting ninety-year-olds who let their age-ravaged hair fall about their shoulders like overcooked pasta, eerily telegraphing the flickers of sexuality that still, apparently, lie beneath.

That's if I make it to ninety after they discover the hideous toxicity of self-tanner, in which I all but bathe.

○

"In my next life, I'm coming back as a beauty editor."

"Do you have any *idea* how good you have it?"

"Hands down, you have the best job in America."

"Now I've seen everything: You get *paid* for doing this?"

I remember the first time I walked into a beauty editor's office. It was delightful and disgusting all at once: shelves upon shelves choking with bath gel, perfume, foundation, lotion, conditioner, lip gloss, eye shadow, cellulite treatments, seaweed serums . . . to one side, a random collection of gifts, from Pucci scarves to yoga mats to novelty chocolates shaped like miniature blow dryers; to another, additional caches of lipsticks, soaps, and shampoos, along with the odd makeup bag and terrycloth robe stuffed in wherever they fit. Every day, cosmetics companies send the beauty editors dozens of packages—my office gets ten to twenty most days—carefully wrapped collections of whatever they're serving up next. We unwrap, and we evaluate.

Whether it's undeserved excess, American overconsumption in general, or blatant female vanity that sends you over the edge, my office contains enough incendiary material to fuel several thousand impassioned protest marches.

Then again, if you've ever waited stammering at a makeup counter while the salesperson wrapped up some overpriced item that you weren't even sure looked good on you (but since

A Big Fat Little White Lie

I don't look like I wear a lot of makeup; neither do most other beauty editors I know. That would be the whole point of makeup, would it not? The idea is you but better: your eyes, but a little bigger, a little more entrancing. Your skin, but with fewer blemishes/wrinkles/blotches. Your lips, but just a tint-y bit more colorful, shiny, and appealing.

On a typical day, my no-makeup look involves:

- self-tanner
- tinted moisturizer
- undereye concealer
- spot concealer
- mascara
- gel eyeliner
- oil-blotting sheets (I've switched from powder)
- If I want to look a whole lot better, I use a little cream blush, but this last step is rarely taken for reasons I myself don't understand
- I also have my eyebrows plucked once a month
- perfume
- Endless reapplications of lip gloss and/or tinted balm. I am not one for a long-lasting lip product. I enjoy putting it on and on and on, and the color and texture I strive for is barely there. I always have at least three imperceptibly different tint/balm/gloss/sheer lipstick varieties rattling around in my bag, so as to be able to constantly change my look without changing my look.

you'd wasted their time and they were so insistent, you bought it anyway), the concept of being able to try on a few colors without a shrill sales pitch attached to it is wildly compelling.

It's like candy, all those little boxes and bottles; a magpie would cock its head and turn its eye so as to take in all the glittering possibilities and probably lose its mind forever right then and there. Beyond my office, though, is the beauty closet, which is about a thousand times worse.

The word *closet* is actually a misnomer. When I worked at *Elle* magazine, the closet was actually an office the size of a large bedroom lined with beauty-item-crammed shelves; now, at *Lucky*, it's three huge walk-in-closet-size closets, again with the shelves, again with more hope in a jar than you can shake a stick at.

There are various cosmetic pioneers who lay claim to the phrase *hope in a jar;* whoever said it was very perceptive. Nowadays, the jars reflect all manner of hopes and dreams, thanks to all the target marketing and brand building and niche identifying: You've got the wrinkle-erasing dream and the clear skin dream, but you've also got much more, from a cleaner earth (Aveda) to a more glamorous life (Chanel) to an edgier, punkier sense of femininity (Stila). You've got the hard-core-city-girl dream (M•A•C, Urban Decay), and the Park Avenue (Estée Lauder), and the dermatologist stamp-of-approval dream that started with Clinique and has recently escalated into Dr. Brandt, Dr. Perricone, and StriVectin SD.

The hands-down most popular dream, cosmetics-brand-wise, is what I like to call the Simone: Simone isn't real, she's an imaginary, dewy, health-exuding French girl. Simone is maybe nineteen, spends a lot of her time naked in spa-like settings, and when she speaks she purses her plummy, puffy lips to say the word *pure*—or, because she's French, it comes out "puuurrrrh." If you want to convince people to buy skin care of any sort, Simone is the woman to sell it to them: Clarins, Lancôme, Chanel, L'Oréal, Remède, Sothys, Darphin, Yves Rocher, Caudalíe, they're all selling you a Simone. The accent in Estée imbues the Estée Lauder brand with lots of Simone. Simone is why there's French on the back of the Origins bottle, the Shiseido compact, and the Maybelline lip pencil, despite those brands' respective, utterly un-French pedigrees/attitudes. It's confounding, but it works: Intellectually, I know I don't want to be a French exchange student in any way, but the Simone is wildly compelling nonetheless.

Like fashion, beauty items are an easy way to try on a new identity—like a kind of costume. As in fashion, some of the options are ridiculous and some are fantastic; at the very least, trying everything on can be a lot of fun. The beauty closet is like a giant costume box full of potential identities that are otherwise under heavy guard from smiling, heavily made-up salespeople armed with perfume spritzers.

The freedom to sift through all the possibilities without having to deal with the "Fries with that?" advisers—with all their advice about what you need and what you don't and what they're supposed to push on you that month—is enough to make most people's heads spin. People tend to freeze up when the door to the beauty closet is finally opened: What to look at first? Who to be?

I get between fifty and two hundred products a day (each package usually contains numerous items), some of them new, some of them just reminders, some of them gorgeous and innovative, and most of them just some dull cream purporting to moisturize some portion of your body, often wrapped up in an equally uninspiring package. The good stuff goes into the closet—either to be photographed for the magazine or to be saved as gifts. The less-interesting stuff goes straight onto the office help-yourself giveaway pile—the place where the fash-

The Fungible Truth

- Many eye pencils come from the same factory in Germany (though everybody's got their own secret formula, some more fabulous than others).
- Sometimes, it's just all about the packaging. In some cases, drugstore brands are better; in some cases, department-store ones are. This is not to discount the power of a good package: If the more glamorous-looking moisturizer makes you feel prettier, that's half the battle right there, isn't it?
- Along similar lines, some things are pricey simply because people want to buy something pricey. When I worked at *Unique Homes,* a luxury real estate magazine, certain fancy houses were in places where they had no neighbors—so no real basis for what their price should be (on some deserted coast in Mexico, ranches way up somewhere in Wyoming, private islands, that sort of thing). So they'd advertise the property at $9 million one month, $29 million the next, $17 million the next. And the cheapest didn't always win: It was all about finding the price that someone wanted to pay. The same principle applies to beauty products. They make $450 eye creams and $60 pots of lip balm because somebody wants to pay exactly that much.
- Nothing from the cosmetics counter is going to erase your wrinkles; it might "reduce the appearance," but that's a different thing.

ion editors put the mismatched socks and the discontinued necklaces; the design editors, the oddly patterned pot holders; and the beauty editors, the shade of nail polish that didn't make it into the article.

The thing that constantly amazes me is there's a market for even the most cretinous, obvious, ridiculous, straight-to-the-giveaway-pile items. The world is full of statistics about how many small businesses fail and how likely it is that the restaurant you're opening will be out of business in three years, but the reverse is true of beauty products. I've seen beauty companies go out of business, but relatively few of them, to be honest. The really good ideas are rewarded with zillions: Somewhere near her mansion in the Steven Spielberg/Kate Capshaw sector of the Hamptons, makeup artist Bobbi Brown docks a boat with the name *TYLL* (*Thank You, Leonard Lauder*—Lauder's being the company that bought hers); Jeanine Lobell, the makeup artist who created Stila, told her husband, Anthony Edwards, he could quit being Dr. Green (on *ER*) when she sold *her* company to Lauder. Roxanne Quimby, the woman who created Burt's Bees, bought the largest piece of land ever sold in the state of Maine (happily, so it could be preserved forever rather than logged or built on) with the proceeds from her business; hairdresser John Frieda was already a wealthy man when Jergens bought his ten-year-old hair care company for $450 million.

While they're busy making their millions, whatever they send that's truly irresistible goes straight into my bag; if I love it as much as I think I'm going to love it, we call in a new one to photograph. It's exactly like shopping, except the mistakes don't cost money and the salespeople are much less withholding.

So I do love my job. What I love most, I think, is that it's impossible to take seriously. So much of it is inane and ridiculous and silly. My beloved shrink tries valiantly to float a "but you're helping all these women feel better about themselves" argument every so often, but you know, I've got a cousin who sits in front of a microscope all day, helping find cures for pediatric cancer.

Me, I ponder lipstick. There are shining pots of ruby gloss, sheer washes of cheek stain, velvet black sweeping lashes. I'm surrounded by mountains of face cream and shampoo—certainly not all of it beautiful—but somehow it speaks to me.

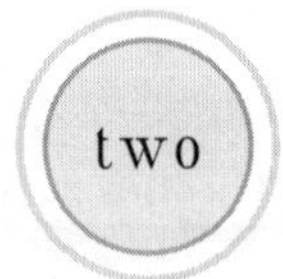

Everybody Loves Beauty (Except When They Hate It)

One of the reasons I love my job is that all people relate to it. I wrote about architecture and interior design when I started out in magazines: While many care deeply about what color the carpet is, many do not.

Everybody loves beauty products. Even if you think you know nothing about them, or even if you think you hate them, you actually know plenty about them and, in fact, have several of them that you love. You have major opinions that lie barely beneath the surface. Women who modestly/moralistically claim to "never use all that beauty stuff" are big Clinique ladies, usually with a healthy helping of Neutrogena to go with. I know this because I've looked in their bags, and I've seen what they lunge for at beauty giveaways (more re that shortly).

There's just *something* about a beauty item: It won't hurt you, it won't make you fat, it doesn't require any sort of emotional investment or exchange of bodily fluids, and it's

A.G.'s Lipstick Corollary

A brilliant editor of mine once discovered this incontrovertible law of nature: Any two random lipsticks you've ever bought—any—when combined, will always be flattering, no matter what your skin tone.

pretty much there just for your pleasure. *And* it could potentially make you look better. A deep green sage bath gel in some unassumingly simple glass bottle, or a cream claiming to painlessly erase wrinkles will have even the most adamant antibeauty operative circling around it like a bear at the zoo that's been presented with a new hunk of raw meat.

Fran Leibowitz (neither modest nor moralistic) once insisted that there was no point in my interviewing her for a beauty story because she *never* used beauty products. It's true that Fran Leibowitz is resolute in her antiglam, antifemme style statement, from her Groucho Marx eyebrows to her Brooks Brothers button-down shirts. But a few sentences later she explained her personal system involving switching among six different kinds of shampoo, day by day: "How else could you tell it was working?"* I don't care how butch/macho you are, there's simply no escaping a beauty moment.

People have such issues with being perceived as vain. The

*I myself believe in an abbreviated version of this theory: There's a single, fantastic shampoo—Phytojojoba from Phyto, for dry and damaged hair, despite the fact that my hair is oily and relatively undamaged—that makes my hair look infinitely better than any other. But I have to keep a few other shampoos around; that way, I make sure the original one remains superior in every way.

Famous! And Perfect!

Next time you open up an article on your favorite female celebrity, count how many words it takes the writer to get to the part where he or she casually mentions "and not wearing a scrap of makeup," "her radiant face completely devoid of makeup," "her beauty amplified by the total absence of makeup." I have yet to read an article about an actress that leaves out this head-exploding detail. When I go to heaven, I'll open up my *Vanity Fair* and there will be articles on Keanu Reeves, Anderson Cooper, and Bill Clinton, all of them with a "he looks just as gorgeous without his makeup" refrain in the first paragraph. What, it's a huge character flaw that Charlize Theron puts on a little mascara before she meets the *In Style* reporter?

worst are the nine trillion models/actresses/socialites who credit their stunning beauty to "the big bottle of water I carry with me always."

But isn't the moment that the severely depressed person picks up a hairbrush, or the cancer patient the tube of lipstick, supposed to be the physician's tip-off that the person's finally pulling out of it? In war-torn countries, black markets always thrive on cosmetics; soap is right up there with sugar and flour on the list of things people hoard first when times get tough. I'm not advocating that more time or money be spent preening and grooming, but it does seem crazy to have such a complex over it.

Maybe that's the French woman thing, the sexy secret everyone's always theorizing over: Maybe French women simply don't feel guilty about being a little vain.

Many have argued that a revulsion of vanity and indeed of women themselves is what powers some of the enormous rage behind the antifur movement. I personally think fur is foul and disgusting (except on its adorable, rightful owners; I have to qualify this statement, though, and own up to the fact that I think other people look wildly glamorous in it), but why is leather more morally acceptable? Why don't they throw blood at construction workers with those enormous clunky boots or (male) captains of industry with their tightly laced $800 John Lobbs? For that matter, why aren't they out there in front of the grocery store screaming at the people with the two-for-one broiler coupons?

There's a movement that's remained sort of nascent throughout my career to ban wearing perfume in public places (primarily public meetings in Berkeley, California) that seems similarly tinged with misogyny. Practically everything we encounter is scented in some way, from dishwashing detergent on down (and up), but fancy-lady perfume is a much easier target to sit in judgment of and aim dogma toward. Give these protesters a few minutes alone with the organic-y glass bottle of sage bath gel, and they'll be circling it just like everybody else.

Even beauty products you do actually hate have an enormous power. I would sneak out of my college boyfriend's room—he and his impossibly handsome roommate sleeping off whatever we'd drunk the night before—as the first chink of rising sun flared at the corner of his window. I crept down the hallway, past the other sleeping geniuses (Stanford; I myself had not gotten in), and into the bathroom. In the heavy silence, at last in front of a mirror, I'd get out a grimy tube of oil-free liquid foundation—the words *cover-up* and *base* flashing

Concealer

There are inconsiderate makeup artists who offer the helpful tip that concealer just makes your breakouts more noticeable. These people forget that they work all day with gorgeous models whose acne is going to be airbrushed out before anyone sees it. I understand what they're getting at—that skin-colored peaks and valleys all over your face still telegraph "acne," so you still need to go to the dermatologist. But a little concealer—don't go with layers, though, no concealer/foundation/powder routine—is the perfect thing for the occasional spot. Dab it on (use the driest formula you can find; the wet ones with the sponge tips are useless, in my opinion, and also seem discomfitingly unsanitary) and pat, don't rub, until it—and your acne—disappears.

through my mind like fire alarms bellowing, shaking even the most deep slumbering from their beds—and set about erasing (modulating, deemphasizing) any trace of acne. I'd had the tube since I was about fourteen; I don't remember buying it or even the events that led up to my being driven to buy it, but it reeked of the Longs, or the Payless, or the Hall's drugstore I bought it in, just the same: fluorescent lights, tampons, greeting cards.

I had a flesh-colored concealer stick, too, so worn that the gold lettering on the side had been ground out of existence long before. It had come vacuum sealed to a cardboard hang tag that required enormous effort to penetrate.

Neither of the flesh tones particularly matched my face—or perhaps they did, and the idea of a flesh tone so revolted me that my mind was unable to reconcile the two as being similar in any way. But I put them on, every morning, in secrecy, fully convinced that without them things would simply not go my way.

Beauty products can fulfill an instinctual passion for perfection—an impulse not unrelated to primate grooming behavior, one that has nothing to do with the opposite sex, or even fashion. You, a big, clunky, blotchy human being, have all sorts of imperfections going on, but if your nails have not one shred of cuticle visible, or not one hair is out of place (think of socialite hair or TV anchor hair), or the skin is seamlessly matte and uniform, you feel that in the face of all the chaos, some order has been restored to the world.

Our slow-moving, overweight science teacher in seventh grade, the unfortunately named Mr. Miles, spent all his spare time in class—while we were watching lurid videos about the dangers of VD or dissecting the sex organs of worms and frogs—creating Viking helmets from remnants he obtained at slaughterhouses. *Remnant* is the most sanitized term I can think of for the horns and piece of the head that holds the two horns together. After he'd soaked them in water (there were buckets of bloody water with little horns bobbing in them dotted all around the classroom), he'd take them out and file them, loudly and carefully, for hours on end. After the filing, it was back in the soak; later, more filing. Eventually, satisfied, he'd take them away and fashion them into helmets, using large ribbons to secure them under the chin.

He would wear the helmets, from time to time, while working on others, and the effect was truly confounding. He was at least four hundred pounds, with thick black hair and pale skin. There was clearly not a drop of Viking blood in him—not that, even had he looked like a Scandinavian Fabio, his behavior would have been any less repellent.

You got the feeling—as you edged past several wobbly-looking, gore-filled buckets and then approached, hesitantly, to ask a question you'd worked every which way to answer without having to actually consult Mr. Miles, trying not to startle him so as to avoid touching any part of him (but especially the file and/or horns)—that the helmets went beyond whatever fashion statement Mr. Miles might have been thinking of. It was something deeply personal and involuntary and grooming related, something that, were it disturbed, might bite you.

A similar over-perfective impulse leaves the victims of overzealous dermatologists and plastic surgeons with preternaturally lineless, wrongly proportioned faces: In their effort to

Are Manicures Necessary?

I thought about it long and hard one night in high school, and I came to a startling conclusion that I immediately shared with all my friends: Manicures are a waste of time. "Like? A boy's going to be into you whether or not you've got nail polish on?" I earnestly explained. Mascara, concealer, lip gloss—those things might get you somewhere, attract someone who might not otherwise be attracted.

So what is it about a manicure? I mean, I'm sure there are men for whom they're everything, but there are men for whom left feet are everything, too. If your average man finds a woman wildly attractive, the lack of a manicure is not going to be a deal breaker. And though it certainly could edge things in your favor (decent, well groomed), even the most perfectly finished one isn't going to get you in the door.

eradicate every last wrinkle, they bulldoze over everything else (or inflate it into odd, cubist contortions).

Manicures are a less alarming, more conventional expression of this sort of perfectionist grooming behavior, if only for twenty-four hours or however long it is until it all chips and frays and smudges into oblivion. Ten fingernails, lacquered like a Chinese cabinet, neat, filed, in place. The world can become a swirling vortex, and you can look down at your hands and think, Order, perfection, control.

Since having children and having my world become an actual swirling vortex, however, I've had about three manicures total. They last about five minutes. I get my perfection kicks with a pedicure, which, unlike the manicure, does I think add a little sexiness to the whole package and generally lasts longer, if only by three days. Because your feet are farther away from your eyes than your hands, I tend to be more forgiving toward chips on a pedicure.

Beauty Giveaway

Whether they're loved or hated, beauty products are like money: They never go on sale, so they have a sort of intrinsic value that speaks to people on some very basic level. At *Elle*, we used to have beauty giveaways, where we'd put out all our excess merch on a conference table and let people have at it. Unfortunately, such an arrangement brings out the ugliest aspects of human nature in about five seconds flat. Those famous experiments when they made the college students divide into guards and prisoners? And had to stop the experiment because the guards quickly devolved into sadists? The

Why Beauty Products Are the Best Presents

1. They're personal, but not too much so (cucumber-mint shower gel—what's not to like and who's not to like it?).

2. The person thinks of you every time he or she uses them, which in many cases turns out to be quite often. (I've always been a big proponent of giving a man you have a crush on either shampoo or shaving cream; not only will he be reminded of you every day, but it'll be at a time when he's a little dreamy, potentially more impressionable, and, perhaps most critically, naked.)

researchers could've gotten to their we're-all-immoral-at-heart results much faster had they thought to throw a few beauty products into the mix: the normally friendly co-workers elbowing one another to get to the head of the line, glowering and grimacing and baring their teeth at one another like a pack of bottle-tailed raccoons.

The doors open, and even the most respectable, highly paid publishing executives transform instantly into ruthless, murderous WWF brawlers, knocking one another over, grappling, pushing, snarling. To control the mayhem, we began charging a nominal $1 or $5 a product (for charity), so people might consider whether they actually wanted that particular shade of nail polish/flavor of bath gel before they bothered destroying their careers trying to snatch it out of someone else's clutches.

At many magazines, there's also a daily giveaway pile, since there are simply too many beauty products, even to save up for a big giveaway. The daily giveaway consists mostly of the extremely dull or the gallingly ridiculous—blue and green nail polish, noxious perfumes, gels and oils that have already oozed themselves halfway out of their jars—but it all goes anyway, every drop of it, right down to the baffling douchelike preparations that are a challenge to get out on the giveaway simply because no one wants to touch them.

The thing about the beauty giveaway is—well, my whole job is a big beauty giveaway—it's irresistible, even to me. When I started at *Elle*, I went to a party at my then-boss's apartment; I had been told that I'd be shocked at the piles and piles of beauty products, at the sheer level of greed, the pure

Bribing Health-Care Professionals Effectively

If someone's in the hospital or a nursing home, load up on the cheap beauty products. While it's fine to give the patient something, that's not the point: Set a budget, and buy as many nail polishes/lipsticks/lotions/perfumes/ whatever the budget allows, put them all in a big bag, and hand them over for the patient to distribute to his or her caregivers.

Not only will the patient receive markedly more receptive care, but he or she will get the not-insignificant zing of power that comes (I'm speaking from experience here) from being the distributor, bestowing rewards on those who are pleasant, withholding them from those who roll their eyes when you ask to have your bedpan changed.

lack of self-control. And I was, when I stepped into her bathroom (as I'm sure every guest made sure to do that evening), deeply shocked and amused and fully superior.

Of course, my bathroom is now about sixty million times worse. Deplorable, in fact. My poor husband, Gary, survives in a state of constant onslaught, as every corner of our house slowly accumulates more scented candles, soap, and conditioner (these are the three items I have the most deep-seated issues over and can't resist hoarding). My children play with the lipsticks and the face creams, pretending the little tubes and jars are characters in some complex and never-ending epic; one of the first words my daughter India was able to read was Origins ("O-gin"), the label on her shampoo.

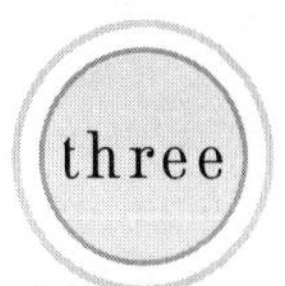

From Ugly Duckling to Swan-ish Ersatz Socialite; or, How I Became a Beauty Editor

Presiding over makeup giveaways isn't exactly the career I'd have predicted for myself (or, come to think of it, even imagined) and certainly not what my parents would have hoped for me. I didn't start out wanting to be a beauty editor; I wanted to be in magazines.

Successful people often seemed predestined to go into their chosen fields; my father, for instance, a prominent evolutionary biologist who studies butterflies, made his first butterfly net with a coat hanger and some cheesecloth at a very tender age. Fashion designers of every ilk always have a story about dressing their mothers or sisters or redecorating the entire neighborhood when they were three; I'm sure Bill Gates's parents have some amusing anecdotes about his nascent Fortran-programming skills (or perhaps his groundbreaking paradigm for lemonade stands that put all the other kids out of business). There's a picture of me reading the newspaper at some early, impressionable age, but that's kind of a stretch, given the only newspaper I was ever involved with was in high school (most of my work there involved interviewing students from different cliques on important style questions).

I did love to write, though beauty never really came up as a topic.

Growing up, I loved beauty products, for the most part—like white bread, chewing gum, and processed cereals, they were not part of the scientist/academic lifestyle I'd been born into. My parents were relentlessly unaware of frivolity in any form: Popular culture and its attendant by-products seemed barely to exist; vanity was not so much reviled as simply unacknowledged.

Like the elf in *Rudolph the Red-Nosed Reindeer* who dreams of being a dentist while the rest of his friends sing carols and manufacture toys, I did not fit in. Moreover, I was keenly aware that without the right accoutrements—any talisman of the culture at large, from the bubble-shaped juice glasses stamped with the Oakland Raiders logo we got for free at the gas station to the zingy copy on the back of the macaroni and cheese box, was wildly compelling—I was not going to fit in with the "normal," glamorous Others, either.

We were not normal people; of this I was positive. Though we lived in a normal tract house (the now-stylish Eichlers of Palo Alto) with a normal postage-stamp yard, our weekends were spent—without exception—hiking, camping, or chasing butterflies up enormous hills. Our summers, while the rest of the *normal* Californians did their beachy, pool-y thing, were spent ten thousand feet up in the Rocky Mountains at a biological research camp.

My parents and my various stepparents are all scientists; they spend their time in laboratories or outside, canvasing the wilderness. My mother canvases for beauty—the sheer granite cliff with the piñon pine and the deep blue sky, that sort of beauty. My father canvases for patterns in DNA; he leads expeditions in pursuit of the butterflies who possess the DNA, his graduate students trailing behind him as he charges up the side of a mountain, hot on the trail. He runs laboratories full of vetch plants growing in vermiculite, nurturing eggs, caterpillars, and full-grown *colias*, fluttering in the warmth of the fluorescent lights. A butterfly is as glamorous as it gets in the animal kingdom: enormous, gorgeous wings dwarfing the functional body, the delicate tongue unfurling to drink the nectar as it embraces the flower. Of course, that's my perspective: The evolutionary mechanisms deep inside the butterfly are the actual beauty part for him.

I was back at home visiting several years ago; I had breakfast with my father in our bathrobes before anyone else was up. I had an English muffin or something, and he had what he has every morning: He upends a can of tuna on a plate, nestling it between two halves of a burned piece of toast. He pours molasses over the toast, coats the tuna fish in about an inch of ketchup, and digs in. He was explaining a recent discovery and got so excited that he brought in huge transparencies dotted with tiny shapes in four specific varieties: DNA. He showed me the patterns, explained the theory and how he'd proved it, shaking the transparencies in triumph. "This is life!" he was saying, and it is life for him, it is beauty. All the hours in the chemical-scented, fluorescent-lit lab calibrating instruments and jotting down data, hours that would kill me, are wildly intriguing to him, foreplay to something earthshaking and beautiful and utterly beyond my comprehension.

I used to think that the adults spoke a different language when they sat in the living room after dinner, and it's true; except for a few connector words, *the*, *a*, *I went*, it was mostly Latin.

My mother, while she did speak the language, had given up professional science, for the time being. Still, my desires—underwear with lace sewn in rows across the back, dolls, flower-sprinkled dresses—were curious to her, and, scientist-style, she investigated them: "What would make you want something like that?" "What will you do with such a thing?"

When scientists are walking along the trail, you have to stop all the time and marvel at this species of plant or that species of bird. "Oh, *Pieris rapae*," I have to stop myself from noting when one of those white butterflies you see everywhere flies by. "Huhnh—a yellow-bellied sapsucker!" "Look, those are some spectacular alluvial fans at the base of that mountain!"

I couldn't access the information I wanted. Our TV went on only for public television. Our stereo played only classical music.

My enchantment with the normal, the mundane, and the average—I wanted cornflakes! Wonder bread! Juicy Fruit! TV on subjects beyond the undersea world of Jacques Cousteau!—was as strong a drive in me as the enzyme within a plant that enables it to contort itself, even against the force of gravity, in an effort to face the sun.

I got it in what little TV I had access to (the chic of the *Zoom* operatives was mesmerizing) and books, especially books with photographs of other people in them. My favorite books when I was little had photographs—specifically, photographs of other small children—because they afforded me a window onto what "normal" people looked like and how they behaved (if this sounds like fodder for decades of dull commentary that some poor therapist has had to endure, well, there it is). Brochures—with their sales-y, upbeat, completely unscientific promises and their glossy photographs—were of particular interest.

I thoroughly enjoyed my several days in the hospital at age six, despite the Stone Age–y urinary-tract-improvement operation I was in for. The enjoyment was all due to the brochure the hospital sent ahead of time, a brochure littered with pictures of happy, attractive children playing in the large playroom, eating off of their food trays, smiling, and holding hands with the kindly, uniformed nurses. As I actually performed my part in these little moments—the best was accepting the promised postoperative Popsicle from the kindly uniformed nurse—I experienced a kind of belonging, a sense of communion with the outside world that I had really never felt before.

Beauty and Sex

Starved for media images beyond the occasional hospital brochure and episodes of *The Electric Company*, I began to look at actual other people: I developed my first crush in the second grade, on a little boy named Eddie with a congenital heart defect who had to go in for open-heart surgery. He told us about it in show-and-tell. Sex, death, and beauty: It starts earlier than you think. Then I loved a little boy, J.B., whose father died halfway through the school year. When he got back from the funeral, he, too, had to repeat the whole tragedy in front of the classroom for show-and-tell. (So heartless and un-PC, my school. But after that, Eddie had nothing on J.B.)

Beauty was straightforward enough as it appeared in the opposite sex: a magical sort of appeal that seemed inborn, DNA-dependent. With girls, I found the signals harder to process. Beauty, social success, and outfits all intertwined in a way that was difficult to make sense of.

In fourth grade I fell in love with my first untragic little boy, Erik, who played my husband in *The Lion, the Witch, and the Wardrobe;* I had begun actively aspiring to a life of glamour and had joined the Palo Alto Children's Theater. The boy who played our son (we were a centaur family) had curly hair, so the costume designer insisted that handsome, Nordic Erik and I wear short, curly-haired wigs to match. I blamed the hideous wig, along with the Pan-Cake makeup, along with the curly-haired boy himself, for the fact that my relationship with Erik never went anywhere; the closest I ever got was helping him fold papers for his paper route. As I folded, I spewed vitriol over the curly-haired boy and the indignity of the wigs, but all I got was a mumbled "Yeah" or two and that was it.

○

The years between sixth and eighth grades were the only ones in which I abandoned my drive for beauty/normalcy. Un–*Reviving Ophelia*, I resigned myself to ugliness and embraced my eccentricity. The specific reasons for this break remain a mystery to me: I changed schools just before sixth grade, just as my parents' marriage was disintegrating and puberty was starting to hit. These three factors add up to something, especially the marriage part, but plenty of children weather similar situations with many fewer visible scars.

Just before sixth grade, the family moved from our Palo Alto Eichler into a sprawling redwood house on campus. My little sister and I were initially thrilled. Not only would we each have our own room, there was a huge playroom attached, all of it at the far end of the house, away from the adults. We were chagrined to learn that our grandparents were moving in as well and that they'd be leveling that part of the house to build their own. We got a tiny guest bedroom split by a hard-to-move sliding door. You'd go to slam your door behind you and find yourself wrenching at this huge slab of wood that wouldn't budge without Herculean effort; you'd decide you wanted some privacy and everyone in the living room would jump, swivel their heads, and stare, startled by the tremendous noise a successful door-pulling generated.

Perhaps from all my years watching *Masterpiece Theatre* on PBS, I became a bit of an Anglophile. I began addressing people with an "-ington" attached to the end of their names—Laurington, Dadington, etc. My grandmother, Gramie (née Gramington), was the only one who indulged me. "Greetings, Gramington," I would say when I went back to her end of the long dark redwood house.

"Greetings, Jeanington," she would reply.

Everyone else refused to acknowledge it. "Hello, Jean," they would sigh.

The puberty thing really stank, because I was obsessed with gymnastics, and suddenly I no longer resembled my idol, Olga Korbut. I would practice the balance beam—in my red leotard—on the fence just outside my grandparents' window. It was about the right height and width; there were great rosebushes twined underneath it. I arched into walkovers and pointed my toes and hopped and skipped as professionally as I could. The spectacle of my newly hormone-infused (I think of those self-basting turkeys) body twisting and flipping awkwardly around on the fence was doubtless what sent my grandmother into action. I can see her coming to the window and watching me, then calling to my grandfather in her high-pitched voice, "Ral-lph!" and pointing out at me. "She needs a bra, doesn't she?" she'd say to him, and he, squinting—he suffered from retinitis pigmentosa and at that point had a 5 percent field of vision—agreeing.

"Well, yes, Lois, why don't you get her one?"

Gramington bought me a bra at the drugstore when she was out shopping—actually several of them, in slightly different styles. They came in slim boxes about the size of single-serving cereal containers, imprinted with photographs of "normal"-looking teenage girls that I stared at for hours. The bras themselves were unpleasant, but what could I do? The gauntlet had been thrown down.

One small victory was that I was allowed to watch the not-on-PBS *Little House on the Prairie.* All those Melissa girls, tumbling in the covered wagon with their long, silky hair and their petticoats. For Halloween, I convinced my mother to make me a "Laura" costume: She made a long, printed calico dress complete with a matching bonnet.

Once the red, flower-speckled bonnet was on, I did not take it off for an entire year. I did not remark upon it, or pretend to actually *be* Laura in any way, and the world responded in kind: I don't remember anyone ever commenting on it. My mother, bewildered as she was by my dolls-and-lace-underwear lifestyle, did not seem to find it out of character.

It was a big bonnet—it was not that no one noticed it. It hid my face, it distanced people; it functioned not unlike blinders on a horse in a busy street. Unsurprisingly, I made few friends at my new school; oddly, though, no one but the very lowest of the weirds bothered to tease me about it.

Bad Hair Day

Though I jettisoned the bonnet the summer before seventh grade, things got worse: My parents did get divorced, the unwelcome hormones were clearly there to stay, I started junior high, and I traded in the bonnet for a refusal to brush my hair. I developed enormous knots, which my junior high compatriots teased me about relentlessly. They were also eager to ridicule my compulsion to save every single one of my used lunch bags, still with the crusts and the apple cores, in my locker; every time I opened it with the key that I wore around my neck on a crocheted pendant, the balled-up paper bags would come tumbling out around me like floodwaters escaping from a burst dam. It was rough, that year.

But even as I shuffled about in my unkempt Toughskins, tangles exploding off the sides of my head, I carried in my pocket the Lip Smackers that all the other girls had (Bubble Gum made me feel, with great relief, part of the mainstream—everybody had it—while Watermelon, to my mind, was a less expected, more sophisticated, sexy-in-a-natural-way sort of option), latent, underground.

While I was attracted to the perfumy shampoos you could smell on someone's hair hours after you'd washed it, and the suntan lotions that promised the dramatic tan lines, I held few illusions about them. They were, for the moment, at least, for other people. I skipped past the beauty articles in the magazines—for the most part, mind-numbing lists of different lipstick shades that rarely related to the model's picture beside them or ways to twist your hair into shapes that would look good only if you were, in fact, that hot girl in the picture.

The magazines themselves, on the other hand, were the thing. I started with *Dyno-Mite!*, which pictured *Zoom*-like kids doing various education-disguised-as-entertainment sorts of things, and moved swiftly to *Seventeen.* I studied them, the beautiful, lucky models with their big teeth and silky hair, gobbling healthy treats and laughing through sexy water fights on the lawn, but I harbored no illusions about ever being like them. The days of aspiration, of fulfilling the hospital brochure promise, were over forever, it seemed.

The First Makeover

But the summer after eighth grade, my perennial Rocky Mountain summer crush, the popular and gorgeous Kevin, who lived in Kansas during the year, was sitting on the steps with me, and he finally sighed and said, "Jean, you should try to be popular. It's a lot more fun." He continued as I regarded him silently. "Like, you don't have to wear that weird tie-dyed T-shirt, and you don't have to never brush your hair. You could pretend to be normal. You might even be kind of cute."

Armed with that single Pygmalion gesture, I returned home from the summer and set about a swift makeover. I called my friend (one of two) Sharon and told her what Kevin had told me. There was a long pause on the other end of the phone; I waited for her to hang up the phone and call our other friend, with whom she'd team up against me forever. I held my breath. "Um," she said finally, "that could really work." We developed the concept further: We would pretend to be new.

Only those who have been as outcast and irrelevant as we were can see the potential in such an idea. "Surely you'd be recognized!" would be any normal person's response. We knew the truth: Not one of our classmates would be able to pick us out of a lineup if their lives depended on it. We had spent the previous two years being completely invisible, and now we were going to cash in.

We brushed our hair and went to the mall for a few key items: French-cut T-shirts from The Limited, Kissing Potion rollerball lip gloss from the drugstore, kohl pencil from the Lancôme counter in Macy's. The clothes make the man, as they say. Sharon had an advantage—her mother's credit card—but I made do. I had allowance money, and Grandma Helen (the relative from whom I inherited the striving-for-glamour gene; she wore perfume and lipstick, had several furs, and referred to her suitcase as "my grip") conveniently came to visit: Clearly relieved that at least someone in the family was like her, she took me to the mall and bought up many of the items I'd fallen in love with.

We also jettisoned the final identifying factor that might have given us away: our other junior high friend. "She's weird," I said to Sharon.

"She's, like, totally strange," Sharon agreed. The truth was that our other friend was markedly less weird than either of us. She already had the French-cut T-shirts and the lip gloss. She had blond hair. Her parents even belonged to a country club.

But three was a crowd, a recognizable crowd, and it wasn't going to work. It was very *Mean Girls/Lord of the Flies/Heathers;* we did it without so much as a bat of an eyelash. I dropped her like my pair of ill-fitting Toughskins, and I never looked back.

We arrived on the first day of high school, completely and utterly New Girls. The wardrobe and makeup helped, but such was our previous weirdness/invisibility that the "new" ploy worked spectacularly, and we were assimilated into the general—even popular—mainstream. Sharon quickly became a head cheerleader and I got myself onto the student council; success at last.

Not that I was suddenly pretty. At no time was I under the impression that the superhot girls were in on some fabulous secret I'd somehow missed. You'd see Beth Davis sunning herself on a redwood park bench (Northern California) in her green bathing suit, hoping to get a little more color in time for cheerleader tryouts, and you wouldn't wonder what shampoo it was she used or what lip gloss she was wearing. No bottle of perfume was going to buy you that future. But I was a little more beautiful, I felt, for my appropriated normality, outfits and all.

Like other teenagers, I cut out pictures of skinny fashion models and pasted them on the refrigerator, despite the fact that I weighed about two pounds at the time. I remember the perfect curve on one model's legs as she crossed them, reclining in her seamless white bikini. If I looked like that, the world would be my oyster, men would fall at my feet, etc., etc.

Perhaps unlike other teenagers, I took the rest of the information in the magazines equally seriously. When I was about fourteen, I started reading *Mademoiselle* (you finish with *Seventeen* at about twelve or thirteen; graduating to magazines

Could You Be Better Looking?

Not that I wouldn't ecstatically accept a ten-pound weight loss and a lifetime guarantee of perfect, glowing skin, but at the end of the day, I'd still be me. While it is technically possible to completely disguise yourself with overdone makeup and/or plastic surgery (an editor of mine once sagely wondered, "Why is it more desirable to look oddly shiny and tightened than wrinkled? Both looks still trumpet 'age' "), less drastic "look better" strategies will still leave you, in the end, looking basically like yourself.

If you can get past—or perhaps embrace—that reality, yes, I think the right haircut, or some knockout mascara, or even a nose job, I suppose, can make a difference. For me, the two indispensible, desert-island beautifiers are a bottle of self-tanner and a pot of undereye concealer. On somebody else it might be a dab of blush or, politically incorrectly, a little Botox. I guess the "dab" and the "little" are the point here. Little things—the sort of change where people ask you, "Did you get a new haircut?" or, "Were you just on vacation?"—can make you look better, but they're not going to erase you. On the other hand, if you're filled with self-loathing in the looks department, no amount of improvement short of something very ugly (fill in the Michael Jackson/Jocelyn Wildenstein/Tammy Faye blank here) is going to satisfy you; you've got to pick up your self-help books and start channeling some embarrassing body-acceptance guru. But again, yes, you could be better looking.

aimed at twenty-five-year-olds is wildly empowering) and happened upon a story in which worldly twenty-five-year-olds recounted the amusing/cautionary/triumphant tales of losing their virginity. I read and reread the article, committing it at least partially to memory. Every time I found myself with the opportunity to lose my virginity, I imagined myself as one of the girls, telling her story, hoping it would be good enough to be included in the article. All the sex talks in the world could not have provided a better form of contraception.

Perhaps I seemed distracted, in the heat of the moment, with Tony Cardoza or Jeff Marth breathing down my neck, as I weighed the important questions in my head: Was it impossibly romantic? Was it somehow memorably funny? Was he so cute or something in his biography so compelling as to get past the editors' exacting requirements? I was eighteen—an age I think most parents and non–Pat Robertson sex educators would be more than happy with—when I finally hit on a potential sexual experience that finally qualified.

Perhaps even more embarrassing, I chose my college—University of Colorado—not, as I told everyone, because I liked Colorado, but because on those annoying subscription cards that fall out of magazines, the return address is always "Boulder, CO 80203." I naturally concluded that all my favorite magazines were produced there and that I'd quickly land a glamorous internship. When I did land an internship at some sort of book publisher, I remember craning my neck around the business park it was located in, sure I'd eventually find the signs pointing me to *Vogue*, *Glamour*, and my still-beloved *Mademoiselle*.

I did finally get an internship doing advertising, which I felt was close—in *media*, at the very least: At home for the summer in Stanford, I created a campaign for the Corner Pocket, the on-campus frozen yogurt and pizza stand. "Sink one in at the Corner Pocket!" said one. "Rack up your favorites at the Corner Pocket!" promised another. The ads appeared in the *Stanford Daily* and were also tacked on post-it boards around the student union; I, or at least my work, was famous at last.

I also actually worked at the Corner Pocket, and it was there, stained with Dutch chocolate yogurt mix and pizza sauce, that I met my future husband, Gary. He was cute, smart, and funny and was undergoing an appealing collegiate obsession with Sartre. He had a punk haircut and a pale blue Dodge Dart. He felt that my pizza-oven-cleaning skills were inadequate, so I would stand back and let him demonstrate the correct way to do it. We've been together ever since.

He decided to chuck graduate school halfway through and become a Dictaphone salesman—an odd choice for someone with a Stanford BA in 1984—but it afforded us the chance to live for a while in Albuquerque, New Mexico, where I learned that we shared an important willingness to sacrifice practicality for glamour: We went shopping for an apartment for the summer and quickly chose the Lakes, a complex that featured a pool, tennis court, and Jacuzzi, all dotted around a gray-green artificial lake. We of course could no more afford all these amenities than a ticket on the Concorde, but we reasoned that quality of life was paramount. The choice meant going without furniture—literally, our dining table was a cardboard box, and we slept on the (carpeted) floor—but it also meant we could swim and soak to our hearts' content. At least once a week we held a sun-damage-inducing, artery-collapsing marathon we called an "Extravaganza," where we laboriously prepared plate upon plate of tempura and blenders full of piña coladas and trucked them all out to the middle of the complex by the pool to eat, drink, and play Scrabble for hours in the baking hot sun. If that isn't glamour, I don't know what is.

We decided to get married after I graduated. My family and friends were horrified—no one in Northern California gets married before the age of forty. Gary's family and friends were also horrified, the family because my decidedly unreligious background clashed diametrically with their fervent, born-again Christianity. There was the never-spoken-of summer of living together in Albuquerque, perhaps a hint of my penchant for piña coladas, and, of course, the fact that my father taught evolutionary biology. . . . I was a less-than-ideal new family member to introduce around at a church social. His friends, on the other hand, some Bible thumping, others not, didn't approve of my state-school, unintellectual pedigree (was he really about to spend the rest of his life with a woman who couldn't possibly comprehend his Sartre infatuation?).

My father, never one for any sort of big celebration, offered to pay for a honeymoon if we'd just skip the wedding part. But of course, by then I was already deep into the bridal magazines, weighing the relative merits of navy blue and hunter green satin for the bridesmaids' dresses (the ugliness of which—I chose hunter green, perplexingly—still astounds me). There was no turning back.

My mom gave us her ancient Honda Civic as a wedding present, and we headed off to Cincinnati, where Gary had a job, and I soon got one—again, in advertising.

I worked at a minority advertising agency; I was the only white person who worked there. Everyone else was black, with black, very curly hair. People liked me, but they felt sorry for me: It was my hair, which at that time was straight (it became wavy after I had a baby). They'd hear that my husband was out of town again (he traveled a lot), and they'd look at me pityingly and drop a suggestion or two: "Do you . . .

WEDDING TIP #1: Take any formal portraits—bridesmaids, etc.—the day before. (You'll never look at them again, but I guess it's impossible not to have them.) Your mouth gets so tired from smiling on the actual day that you waste all the good smiles on the boring formal ones and end up with a grimace in the happy-fun-reception ones.

WEDDING TIP #2: Take pictures of yourself with the veil on beforehand. Better yet, shop for the veil with a Polaroid. The only pictures I can stand to look at from my wedding are after I've taken off the veil.

ever try hair spray—you know—for volume?" inquired the kindly account executive.

"I wonder, if you *had* a blow dryer," ventured the art director, "maybe . . . you could get your hair to . . ." The whispered tips about mousses and curling irons rose gradually to a roar, and finally I was dispatched to a salon to get a perm. Getting the perm, sitting there with all the chemicals and rods in my hair took forever; it smelled terrible and was extremely expensive. But without that perm, I was never going to fit in.

The results, though underwhelming—I looked disappointingly like myself, except with much curlier hair; it was not one of those transformational moments like a makeover in a magazine—drew a collective sigh of relief around the office. "Honey," the receptionist greeted me on Monday, "that's *a lot* better."

Eventually, after a stint in Ypsilanti, Michigan (I wrote ads for an Ann Arbor radio station), Gary got transferred to New York. I've never been so happy. We moved in with Grandma Helen in Maplewood, New Jersey, and I strode off to the city, ready to make my mark. Dispiritingly, every ad agency I went to explained that I'd need to start as a receptionist, as I was only a year out of college. Did I love advertising enough to start over? I did not.

The Big Time

I had gone into advertising because I found the seriousness of "journalism" tedious and uninspiring (if not illusory, which is another conversation) but found my métier at *Unique Homes*, a luxury real estate magazine where I wrote ads half the time and articles the other half. This was clearly ideal training for writing about beauty: As fashion magazines are supported primarily by their beauty advertising, articles about beauty products are always raves and never probing, critical works.

I worked along in obscurity, getting my fix of glamour wherever I could—my publisher occasionally told tales of his two dates with "Tama," the *Slaves of New York* authoress who was the female embodiment of all that was cool in late-'80s New York; similarly, there was an ad salesperson in Florida who'd gone out with Billy Idol. Every so often I'd be invited to a party myself, something from the industry. I dined out for weeks on the free lunch I had at the Plaza, courtesy of a toilet fixture manufacturer. It happened to be my birthday that day. The sun was shining; I practically skipped along Fifty-ninth Street toward the Plaza, thinking that really, things did not get much better. The hors d'oeuvres contained caviar! The dessert involved petit fours! So what if I had to listen to an hour's worth of toilet-fixture propaganda?

And so what if I had to make up that hour or two of lost

work at the end of the day? We all worked until 10 p.m. every night, anyway, so it took me a while to catch on to and appreciate the biggest downside of the press-lunch thing: You've still got to write your article and get the rest of your work done (in the case of *Unique Homes*, this involved calling the hideous Realtors across the country who you were writing ads for, trying to get their approval on copy that you'd translated roughly into English, only to have them scream into the phone at you to change it back).

I met one of my best friends, Mayer, on a press trip to a vinyl flooring factory in southern New Jersey. I had become an editor at the obscure *Contract Design*, a trade magazine for architects and interior designers, and he held a similar position at the much more glamorous *Interior Design*. It was August and about ninety degrees; the vinyl flooring factory promised to be many degrees hotter. A tour bus pulled up to take us there; Mayer and I happened to sit across from each other and simultaneously slap down the same hot-off-the-presses, six-zillion-page September issue of *Vogue*. We looked up, instant kindred spirits, thrilled to have someone share in the indignity of vinyl flooring factories and the hope that someday, somehow, we would no longer have to tour them. (Mayer now sits a few floors up from me as design editor of *House & Garden*, a fate that would have seemed impossibly grand had it been presented to us there in the tour bus.)

I tried getting interviews for jobs at bigger magazines, but interviews seemed to be solely for people with connections, and I had none. Instead, I began writing articles—mimicking the style of whatever magazine I was aiming for—and sending them in, already finished. All journalism classes will advise you to send magazines queries—proposals for articles that you submit to editors. For me, writing the query takes longer than writing the article. Or it's more stressful, anyway. In any case, it worked: I sent articles in to both *New York* magazine and *Condé Nast Traveler*, and, miraculously, they printed them.

Then I wrote a piece about a makeup artist who had just created a set of lipsticks—an unassuming woman named Bobbi Brown—and sent it in to *Vogue*. They went for it, and my career took its fateful direction (of course, if only I'd instead joined up with Bobbi Brown on the lipstick idea, I'd be writing this book from my yacht).

Once the *Vogue* piece was out, I had a new career. Never underestimate the power of *Vogue*. Suddenly, doors opened, phone calls were returned. Every magazine called me and wanted articles; I freelanced and I freelanced, and I barely slept, I had so much work. People always ask me—especially now that I've got kids and everything—why I don't just freelance. It sounds so easy and relaxing, *free*lancing, but the reality for me, anyway, was that I felt I couldn't say no to anyone, ever. Why would they call you for the next article when you said no the first time? I had no social life and barely a marriage while I freelanced, and I was desperately sleep-deprived.

I started doing a lot for *Elle*. Then a senior editor position came up, and since the editor in chief liked the articles I'd done for them, she was willing to overlook the fact that I had no experience whatsoever in the beauty industry.

The day I started the job at *Elle*, I got so many flowers my office looked like a funeral parlor. Looking at them long and hard, I realized that if I had in fact died, the flowers would not be for me. They'd be for my replacement.

The Bobbi Brown Paradox

The makeup industry still does not fully understand the Bobbi Brown phenomenon. The thinking is—and it's true for most brands—that you've got to have something wildly experimental every month or so at the counter to keep people coming back. The "styles have changed so I must spend some money" theory. This works with skirt lengths (though now, of course, all bets are off), but even skirt-length changes take several years to actually take effect. The sudden imperative for turquoise eye shadow is artificial, A.

B, The other thinking is, the more stuff they pile on you, the more you'll buy. This must be at least partially true, or counterpeople (the industry calls them beauty advisers, which is fine, the way people who go door-to-door selling encyclopedias could fairly call themselves educational advisers) would have quit trying by now.

Somehow, though, Bobbi Brown makes money just making people look pretty and stopping there. Her counters swarm with customers. If somebody makes you look good and doesn't fly into a rage because you want to buy only that one shade of blush, you come back.

When you see drag queens, do they look like they've been to a Bobbi Brown counter? They don't.

Since many makeup companies cannot see past the "Hot Trend!" approach, nor can they imagine not riding their counterpeople to rack up as many items as possible per sale, they're always looking for other ways to explain the Bobbi Brown phenomenon. First, it was her black packaging; then they'd come out with all neutrals. They keep casting about, but so far there's no Bobbi Brown equivalent anywhere.

I wish there were one in fashion. Can you imagine? If there were a true Bobbi Brown in fashion—who never presented short-shorts with a business-suit jacket, for starters, someone whose black pants were cut in the most flattering way possible no matter what, who always made you look good?

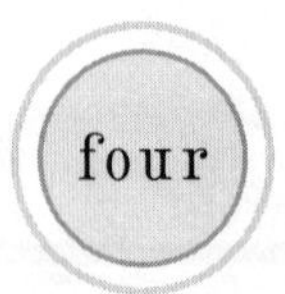

Does She or Doesn't She?: Beauty Tips and Beautiful People

Beauty *advice* is far more problematic than the products. From the drag queeny automaton behind the makeup counter who says you need contouring powder and four separate shades of eye shadow to the magazine articles that employ wild graphics, supermodels, and unendurable puns, all to suggest you wear moisturizer if your skin is dry, most of the people *with* the advice are desperate to sell you something. (Or, in the case of the water "tip," desperate to sell themselves as unvain and thus superior human beings.)

The good beauty advice is the kind you get in the locker room at the gym, when one girl is telling her friend about this amazing new mascara that makes her eyes look five thousand times bigger and doesn't run, and as she goes to pull it out of her bag, every head in the room whips around like Linda Blair's in *The Exorcist.*

Everybody's got a beauty tip, a beauty story. Celebs especially. If you're a journalist and celebrities refuse to re-

The Very Best Beauty Advice I Have for Anyone

Complainers are the worst. The way to tell a talent from a charlatan in any sort of "attractiveness advisory" role—makeup artist, facialist, manicurist, or hairstylist (to whom this rule applies double time)—is that the truly good ones are forever telling you how beautiful you are. The other option, since they must engage with your appearance in some way, is the "you're broken, let me fix you, let me help you cover it all up, you poor thing" ploy or, worse, the strategy of deploring the work of the last beauty expert you've been to ("Who *did* this to you?"). No thanks. Just walk out the door.

The pro-you operatives aren't just obsequious, ass-kissing, money-hungry predators, either. For the most part, a good deal of their talent lies in the fact that they see beauty in many people and use their magic to *play up* that beauty rather than the "this dark lipstick will distract people from your enormous nose" routine of lame behind-the-counter "adviser"—types who jump out at you as you're walking by with a cheerful, "You look like you really need something for your undereye bags!"

veal anything good when you're interviewing them, ask them when they first tried makeup. I guarantee something involving alcohol, drugs, or the opposite sex is the next thing coming out of their mouths, or, at the very least, some unintentionally revealing comment about their family. Ask them if they think perfume has the power to create memories. Suddenly they're giggling and smiling and telling you about the time they slept with that other big celeb at the truck stop in Tallahassee.

The first story *Vogue* assigned me was on nails; the editor sent me for a pedicure at the Warren Tricomi salon. Scavullo, the famous 1970s photographer (any *Cosmopolitan* cover you can remember, that's him) was getting a very careful, shiny manicure in the corner.

I was led to a royal blue love seat perched high above a shining, hammered-copper bowl (very *Sheltering Sky:* You dangle your feet in it as the pedicurist kneels before you and scrubs). Across from me, on another royal blue love seat, was Robyn Byrd, the famous/infamous queen of New York cable porn (she hosted an eponymous, mostly nude interview show). Peeling

Creativity and the Foot

Better to wear your artistic masterpieces on your feet than on your face, I say. There's something about a spray of silver glitter or an adorable miniature daisy that somehow isn't horrifying in a pedicure.

- That said, it takes a lot of time for a pedicure to dry, so you won't be getting another right away, even if money is no object. So think about the shoes you'll be wearing for the next two weeks before you pick a color that will in no way go with your fabulous new sandals.
- White or palest pink is tan enhancing; Chanel Vamp (black red) is by far the sexiest shade, though if it's summertime, the sandal factor needs to be considered; red and hot pink are similar to Vamp in all aspects except they lack Vamp's alterna/sexiness vibe; middle-range pinks always look to me as though the person is experiencing heart trouble and her nails have gone a little blue; corals and oranges are best left for truly tan people, except for the fact that they accentuate leathery skin like no other color, so beware; the Crayola-color colors had their moment about seven years ago and currently transmit a mall-ishness that is the polar opposite of stylishness and intrigue.

her jeans up over her knee to reveal mismatched, well-worn tube socks, Byrd ignored me strenuously, major-celeb style, until she noticed I was taking notes (the pedicurist was making pronouncements about how to tell a good polish from a bad). When she found out I was writing for *Vogue*, she all but sat in my lap and proceeded to compete furiously with the poor manicurist to make the loudest, most definitive pronouncements about the art of the pedicure. "I always get white polish," she confided, smiling her trademark, nasolabial-fold-emphasizing grin and splaying her freshly polished toes for viewing. "The white makes your feet look tan [true enough, I should add], and it's sort of—I don't know—innocent."

The Makeup Tip Defense

Makeup tips are a fine way to defuse envy—perhaps why breathtaking models and actresses are often so hot to dispense them. If I were a gorgeous woman, I'd get myself a pat answer ("Oh, it's my mascara, actually. I was a fucking dog until I discovered it—look! Isn't it great?") and tell the people where to go buy it. The way celebs who take the offensive and try to sell their interviewers something—scientology, saving the children, whatever—escape the truly hard questions by boring the interviewer into wrapping things up quickly.

The idea that the beautiful person has a secret that, if shared, would bestow beauty upon anyone is very, very compelling. Hence the gorgeous models and actresses on the cover of every magazine and hence the women all over the country marching into stores with said covers, demanding to buy the makeup we've put on the models' faces.

My middle cousin, Hannah, is the best-looking person in our family. Beautiful girls are often noted for their "sense of style"—as if somehow the way they put together their outfits were the key to why they look so fantastic. We all coveted Hannah's clothes. She loved these pullover ski parkas called Mother Karens. We were walking in town one day when she was maybe in sixth grade, and high school boys—*high school*—came up.

"Hey, Hannah," said one. "What's happening?"

"Hannah," said another, "where'd you buy your Mother Karen? It's so cool."

Once, Hannah and I went cross-country skiing, and I had to borrow a jacket, and somehow she let me wear one of the Mother Karens. It was freezing and pouring snow, conditions that would normally send me straight to the ski lodge for a day of hot chocolate in Styrofoam cups, but I skied and skied like a

Foolproof Feel-Good Tip

People often ask me if it's difficult to go to photo shoots surrounded by gorgeous, crazily thin, toweringly tall models. My thing is I just don't look in the mirror while I'm at the shoot. This may not work for everyone, but the first time someone asked me the question, I realized that I quite enjoy being around gorgeous models. Something in my admittedly mysterious psyche clicks in when I'm around one and I think, Isn't it great that we're all so skinny and good-looking? The effect lasts all day, until I finally get a glimpse of myself once I'm home and have forgotten about the no-mirrors rule and think, Wow, I had a really rough day. But I comfort myself with the fact that I'm probably tired and I've been looking at skinny models all day.

fiend that day. I was old enough that my hair length had been wrested from my mother's control, so it flowed past my shoulders. Peering out from my now-acceptable hair, inhabiting the Mother Karen, and regarding Hannah in an environment devoid of mirrors, I started to experience—a little, enough, anyway—what it might feel like to *be* Hannah.

How Do I Look?

At the opposite end of the tip spectrum is the idea that you could subvert someone's natural beauty. In high school, Sharon (of pretending-to-be-new fame) would pick me up and we'd go to the Stanford Shopping Center. Shopping with Sharon was fun but also a drag because she had her mom's credit card, so we were not exactly playing on a level field.

The Emporium would, of course, have nothing. We'd cross through to Macy's and look at eye shadow and skin cream. Then we'd eat: Chicken McNuggets with pineapple dipping sauce or Chinese chicken salad.

I had become a connoisseur of the many McDonald's offerings (I think they did a lot of their test marketing in the Stanford Shopping Center location) when I briefly worked there when I was fifteen. Free food, spending money—what was not to like? Until the day the manager suggested I mop the floor out in the dining area. This was a problem because of the tight, high-waisted, excrement-brown polyester pants that were part of the uniform, which, when you were safely behind the counter, could not be seen.

I held my breath, mopped faster than you've ever seen someone mop, praying that no one I knew would happen upon the cringe-ifying sight of me wearing the pants. When I left that night, I left the entire fry-vat-scented uniform crumpled in a heap in the changing room; I never returned.

In The Limited, we'd bring about six zillion things into the dressing room. When Sharon tried something on, when she'd turn to look in the mirror, her entire face would change. It'd be creepy, except everyone on earth does a version of it: mirror face. One normally very sophisticated and feminine friend of mine always turns involuntarily toward the mirror in a three-quarter profile, sucks in her cheeks, and purses her lips like one of the competitors in *Paris Is Burning*. An even more exuberant friend flings his arms in the air with the drama of Madonna in the *Material Girl* video, crossing his wrists, parting his lips seductively, lowering his eyelids halfway, and thrusting his hips out just so, just to look at himself in a T-shirt.

Sharon's version involved cocking her head to one side like a model in a catalog and somehow managing to glance down and then up in a millisecond—very come-hither—and at the same time she'd hunch in with her shoulders and put her hands on her hips. She'd smile-glower at herself longer than you would—if you realized you were doing it.

"How do I look?" she'd say.

Well. Sharon looked good in most things, most of the time. But my answer depended on how truthful I felt she'd been with me on that issue lately.

Sometimes I'd think that something actually did look good on me, and she'd say, "No, don't do it. All wrong." And I'd think, Really? I'd usually try to press for a reason, and if it sounded weak, I'd either try to convince her with the reasons I liked it or I'd put it on hold and come back later with Alisa or Julia and ask what *they* thought.

Did I ever tell Sharon something looked bad on her that didn't? Or that something looked good when it actually wasn't so flattering? I limited myself on those things. Like if she'd done it to me a lot lately, yes. Or if she had like five bags of stuff and I had a package of hair elastics from Woolworth's, OK.

Your friend is supposed to tell you what the mirror can't; is there a worse sort of intimate betrayal? (Especially letting the person walk around wearing something ridiculous because you told her she looked cute in it.) But what you say to the "How do I look?" involves all sorts of internal maneuvering, not all of it reflecting cold, unblinking evil.

My college roommate Susan was very beautiful, and all of us vied to borrow her clothes and makeup. Like the Hannah phenomenon. But her cute boyfriend finally put the kibosh on the practice when she got this incredible yellow sweater. (It looked incredible on *her*; yellow not being the most universally flattering color, I'm sure the rest of us looked awful in it, but you're as beautiful as you feel, right?) The boyfriend would have none of it: She alone was beautiful to him, and he would not have her hallmarks defiled by lesser operatives such as ourselves. (We continued to borrow her lip gloss and shower gel unimpeded, of course—that's the beauty of beauty as opposed to fashion.)

There are some how-do-I-looks that are not true requests for advice. People want you to rubber-stamp the skirt/lipstick shade/short-shorts they're enchanted with. Such a person rarely looks you straight in the eye when asking for the advice; they glance around, hoping against hope. Morality here can be tricky, but I err on the side of rubber-stamping unless the thing is genuinely hideous.

One false move, though, and you run the risk of ruining your credibility. You become one of those people who lets their friend go for their Barbara Walters interview with a big splotch of spinach covering one of their front teeth.

But sometimes you honestly don't know how you feel about a particular look. This is the worst, because the person thinks you know and you're just not saying. I have a problem with this particular scenario and am constantly accused of shadiness and dishonesty as a result. "If I had a gaping ulcer the size of a pumpkin on the side of my face, you'd come to visit me in the hospital and you wouldn't even mention it!" fumes my friend Adam. " 'Oh, what, I don't see anything. . . . Oh *that*, well, I can barely see it. . . .' "

You can not know for a variety of reasons: (1) You hate the entire genre. Your friend is trying on coral lipstick, and you hate coral. Does she look pretty in it? It's hard to get past the fact that you hate coral. (2) The person is impossibly attractive and she'd look hot no matter what she put on. Yeah, you look great in the potato sack and the white gauchos *and* with the green slime sticking to your face. A variant of this is the Grandma Helen phenomenon, where you're blinded by your love for the person.

Grandma Helen always thought I looked great, but she always fell down at another how-do-I-look stumbling block: loving a particular genre. I think I've mentioned about the Dorothy Hamill haircut. You could have the roundest, most unpleasantly featured and chinless face on earth and Grandma Helen would still recommend—with such vehemence as to be fairly termed shrill—the Dorothy Hamill. You could have horrible rosacea and carrot-colored hair and she'd still vote for the tomato-red winter coat. Gary and I lived with her when we first moved to New York; I took the train in every day. Every day, I'd be ready to leave and she'd squint at me critically: Something was not quite right. "You don't look like the other girls," she'd say. I finally got to the bottom of it, and it turned out she was enchanted with the white Reeboks that all the she-lawyers and lady bankers (it was the 1980s) on the train wore until they reached the office and slipped into their pumps. I tried; I could not conscience a Reebok; I bought some other, less offensive sport shoe as a substitute. Finally, I came home one day to find a Reebok box slapped down on the table in front of me.

"I went to the Short Hills Mall today," she said, a challenge in her voice. "I got you something."

Conversely, advice can be too advanced for its intended recipient. I was skeptical when I went downtown one day to see Lauren Hutton's new makeup line: Who needs makeup less than a model? When I stepped into her Ruscha/Schnabel/Clemente-strewn office, I practically said it out loud: At an age when many of her contemporaries are mired in surgical procedures and thickets of foundations and powders (she's sixty or so), Lauren Hutton exudes a pure animal magnetism. She's not just beautiful, she's got an extra portion of aliveness. She certainly doesn't need makeup.

This was, in fact, her point: She got out old magazines and photo shoots of herself, and she contrasted the tarty, overly lipsticked ones with a Barneys ad by Steven Meisel where she gamboled, seemingly clean faced, in a tropical paradise. Both looks involved makeup; only one conveyed the animal magnetism.

She brought me over to her desk and did *my* makeup: concealer/blush/contour/lips—all done with cool, painterish brushes. "It's funny having someone you just met touch your face," she observed. She had some great tricks: One that really made a difference was putting a stripe of concealer down the center of your nose. "It makes it look smaller," she explained, eyeing her handiwork with obvious satisfaction and handing me a mirror. I looked—it's true—like I didn't need any makeup. Brilliant!

Except, though I love her concealer and use it often, I can't do the stripe. It's just too much for me; I feel I need additional training. Lauren Hutton has spent her career watching makeup artists put stripes of concealer down her nose, so she's seen it work over and over, and she knows how to do it. Great advice, too advanced.

I wandered around SoHo for hours afterward, willing someone I knew to appear and remark on how well I looked, so I could laugh self-deprecatingly and murmur, "Lauren Hutton just did my makeup."

Then there's the advice you know is right and you know you're capable of . . . but you refuse to take anyway. All people agree that my pants need to be tighter and I need to wear more eyeliner. But my fear of looking like a slut holds me back no matter how heartily people laugh at my unflattering ways. It has been illustrated to me on countless occasions—by the most talented makeup artists in the world, P.S.—that a little bit of blush makes everyone, including me, look significantly prettier. Do I understand why I won't wear the blush? I don't. I look better with it on, and I never manage to make it happen.

But back to pure, unadulterated lies. Men like to think women reserve their nastiest beauty-undercutting strategies for other women, but this has not been the case in my life, so far.

Before I left for college, my father's (male) graduate students sat me down and gave me a few ground rules: Don't drink too much (we were drinking beer as we had the conversation), etc.

They emphasized one rule above all others: DO NOT DATE ANYONE ON YOUR FLOOR AT THE DORM, EVER. This seemed easy enough. Especially after I saw the less than appealing array on our floor; no chance. Unfortunately, one day the glazed-eyed-hippie one got a haircut and was suddenly, inexplicably cute. For about two seconds, we were in love. Naturally, a sick, wrong, and humiliating breakup ensued. "I hate you. . . ." I can still hear him, taking a drag from an enormous bong, spilling it on the floor, and laughing gutlessly as he himself fell into the pool of bong water. "You are so fucking—*uncool.*"

And there we were, as the graduate students had warned me, stuck together on the same floor for the rest of the year (it was September). The only solution was to become "friends." A month later, my "friend" had two Halloween parties to go to. "I need two costumes," he whined (he wasn't the sharpest knife in the drawer to begin with, and his judgment was further clouded by a constant stream of psychedelics).

I obliged with a cheerleader costume for the first party, complete with a full face of makeup and awful pink lipstick. He returned the next day, dejected. "Every girl I tried to talk to at the party walked away from me," he said.

I made a sympathetic, surprised expression. "Really? I can't imagine why."

"Well. I need a new costume for tonight." I came up with a concept he embraced enthusiastically: a nerd! He thought it was hilarious.

We put him in a button-down and a tie, and he regarded himself in the mirror, wildly amused and confident he would attract scores of women with his handsome yet ironic look. I then combed gobs and gobs of pink, noxious conditioner through his hair. "Nerds have greasy hair," I explained. Then I spent close to an hour creating fake "acne" out of concealer and lipstick; I sent him off assuring him how realistic and great it all was. Unsurprisingly, there was no action for him at that party, either.

Hot Models

It's true, though, there is that "we hate her" girl thing. It leads only to unhappiness on all sides. My beautiful friend Jennifer is not just beautiful, she is also tall and very thin like a model. Almost every single time we've gone into the steamroom at the gym, some disgruntled woman will blurt out, "Does she eat?" at me, as if Jennifer were not sitting there, naked besides, in front of her. "Don't you just want to kill her?"

So models do have it rough, I suppose. The guilt over all that envy. Don't you just hate her? I wonder what she'll look like when she's old and fat? It's gross. The beautiful people who try to make room for such reactions fare the worst, in my opinion. You know that look, "I know I'm beautiful, please let's get past it, I'm sorry, let's just move on"? That particular expression makes a person as invisible, bland, and annoying as a beautiful person can be. Like she might get to be a talk show host at best, but she's never going to be a movie star.

Or she could end up selling skin cream. Not that there's anything wrong with getting a contract and posing for an ad campaign, but there's a point where it turns and the model/actress takes everything too seriously and starts insisting the cream she stands to make zillions off of is the reason she looks the way she does.

Big cosmetic companies generally seem to understand this offensive-if-it-goes-too-far conflict of interest and train their spokesmodels, celebs or no, to mention their favorite items without going overboard. The independent spokesmodel who's partnered with some chemist to create her own, revolutionary line is typically less restrained. Especially wrong if the model's already sliding down the slippery slope of being over, and then the desperation is all around you, mixing in with the sales pitch and making it all the more uncomfortable.

A famous supermodel was once introducing her new skin care line. We were sitting on white sofas, facing each other; the products were on a table between us. There was a long, silent moment. "The products look great," I said.

"This is weird," she said in a panicked, vaguely threatening tone, and waving her publicist over.

"Um, I'm used to being interviewed?" she said half to the publicist and half to me. "Like they ask me the questions and I answer? I'm not used to, to . . . *presenting*."

"But that's what we're doing here," explained the poor publicist. "You're presenting your line. You tell the editor why you developed the products, what's in them—"

"OK, I get it!" she snapped, and whirled back to me, resigned to her fate. "The signs of aging . . ." blah blah blah. It's rough, as I say.

My favorite model endorsement moment was at a huge fragrance launch at the top of the Empire State Building. The company had flown in editors from all over the world, spent zillions of dollars on the fragrance, the new supermodel to endorse it, renting out the Empire State, etc. They had lunch, they had music, they had entertainers, they had announcements. Then the supermodel got up to take questions. "How do you like the fragrance?" asked some enterprising young reporter. What a ridiculous question! Why, it smells fantastic! Out of this world! In fact, exactly like $6 million or whatever I got for endorsing it, sir!

The model stammered for a moment and then said—clearly, into the microphone—"Well, I haven't actually smelled it yet, but I plan to."

Natural Beauties

Whether stupidity undermines beauty remains—and will remain, as long as humanity roams the earth—a subject of important debate (short-term, one night or so, it certainly troubles most people very little). Just as models exhibit the same incredible differential in intelligence as the general population, there's a similarly vast spread regarding how they actually look in person. Some models—even major supermodel types—do appear truly unremarkable, even downright ugly, until you see a picture of them. And others are just simply gorgeous, gorgeous, gorgeous, nonstop. It's not necessarily a question of with makeup or without, most of the time; some otherwise not-hot people just happen to look gorgeous in front of a camera. The all-gorgeous-all-the-time ones—Christy Turlington is particularly amazing—really are incredible to look at. But the others—the only-in-a-picture ones—help keep things in perspective.

Researchers have studied what makes a person beautiful quite extensively. There's the symmetry thing—sadly, as my features correspond in only the vaguest way from one side of my face to the other. In theater class in high school, they made us take two identical Polaroids of ourselves, cut them in half, and glue the two same-halves together. The result, for me, was one attractive face and one hideous face. I think we were supposed to remember so we'd know which side to be photographed on once we became famous movie stars. What sticks in my mind is only the fact of the appalling dichotomy, the horrifying *Sybil* moment.

If you're female, your features are most ideal if they resemble a baby's: big eyes and lips, tiny chin.

And then there's the ratio thing. Over the years, I've polled every man I ever knew, relentlessly, about the importance of face vs. body. I just can't believe body is more important than face for men. But they all consistently say the same thing. Would you rather sleep with a woman with a beautiful face and a so-so body or a woman with a beautiful body and a so-so face? I ask. They all choose so-so-face woman. It's incomprehensible to me. Gary and I went to a party where the hostess was the skinniest, most artificially enhanced sixty-five- to seventy-year-old you've ever seen. Her poor face was a windblown Halloween mask; her forward-facing breasts hovered unmovingly above the tray of hors d'oeuvres she carried; her tiny ant legs gripped the leopard-print carpet on spindly Jimmy Choos. She looked insane.

"So that wife was pretty hot," Gary said as we drove home. I looked at him in disbelief. "I mean, for her age," he said. "Her body looked pretty good, anyway."

The right ratio—I don't know precisely what it is—of breasts to hips to waist, perhaps, it's all somehow ab-related—sets them off, and they see nothing else, the researchers tell us. Stick in a little extra padding, or stick on a face that leaves a little to be desired, because they won't care. They just want to

Models and Distorted Body Images

If the endless protests were true, and the media images of skinny models were truly responsible for the plague of anorexia and bulimia, then what about the huge increase in obesity that's mirrored our society's increased fascination with—and indeed the increased proliferation of—media images of skinny models? Most people blame the food industry for the obesity and the magazines for the anorexia. Something doesn't quite add up.

see the correct ratio. It's like those poor baby monkeys they forced to attach to the chicken-wire mothers. As long as the form even vaguely follows function, men will respond. It doesn't matter whether the blush you used was a powder or a cream.

There's a ratio for men, too, and I don't know precisely what it is, either. I don't need to: You know it when you see it, right?

Ever since the studies about the ratio came out, though, I feel better about my appearance, not worse. My abdominal area—which I'd previously despaired over—now seems so powerful, attractiveness-wise, that it feels like a suddenly discovered asset.

It turns out you can be cellulite-free, gleaming from head to toe, and physically perfect in every way, and you're still just as likely to be cheated on, dumped, and disappointed as the rest of humanity. One of my womanizing bosses taught me this inadvertently, as he screwed over top, won't get out-of-bed-for-less-than-$10,000-a-day supermodel after supremely-gorgeous-most-sought-after-woman-in-the-world supermodel, delighting in the trail of gorgeous misery he left in his diminutive, sixty-or-so-year-old wake.

He married one supermodel and famously cheated on her. (His very graphic accounts of precisely how it all happened were detailed to a British tabloid; his comments were too specific to make it into the papers here.) One unlurid detail was that the supermodel he was cheating with made a large stencil of the shark tattoo on his shoulder; she spray-painted out a path of stencilled sharks, leading from her door to the building several blocks away that he shared with his supermodel wife.

In the end, I think money buys more happiness than beauty does, despite all the cautionary tales. (Warhol agrees with me on this.) Except that if you've got money, you can fund a Sisyphean quest for beauty that rarely ends well. The most attractive man I know is forever asking me about jaw implants—fortunately for him, he's remained short on cash, so he hasn't yet been able to rush out and destroy what nature gave him.

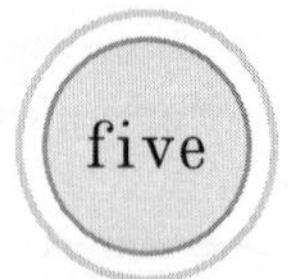

Free Lunch

An enormous part of the beauty editor job involves going out to lunch—and breakfast, high tea, drinks, dinner, and everything in between. And while endless rounds of Le Cirque and Jean Georges sound fabulous, rest assured: Any way you slice it, there still is no free lunch.

There's the phenomenon I mentioned earlier, where you go to the three-hour lunch and return to your desk with a three-hour deficit in your workload. No one at the office is ever terribly sympathetic to your overworkedness, since they got neither a fancy lunch nor a big bag of beauty products. Then add in the fact that most beauty editors end up going not just to a lunch, but to several events, every day (breakfast, lunch, tea, drinks, dinner, etc.). And that most of the lunches, events, etc., are not optional. If a beauty editor were to avoid them—if she always sent another editor from the beauty department in her stead—the cosmetics companies who throw them would eventually grow mightily displeased. Avoiding that situation is a large part of the beauty editor job—not as important as coming up with ideas, articles, and visuals the readers love, but close.

There's not a fancy restaurant I haven't been to, but at most of them, I've been sitting across from a reasonably pleasant person whom I'd never otherwise choose to speak with, all things being equal (and who'd probably otherwise never choose to speak to me, all things being equal). It used to pain me deeply when the person would inevitably pull out a bagful of products right there: Invariably, the person produced a huge, technical-looking bottle of lotion or a collection of twenty-four different lipsticks, each of them carefully opened up and displayed on the table like so many miniature but phallic soldiers, bursting with brilliant oranges and fuchsias, creams, mattes, and pearls.

There's a Darwinian pecking-order thing that's at its most extreme at an expensive New York restaurant; if you so much as blink when a huge celebrity passes by your table, you lose many points. If you crane your neck to see, say, Henry Kissinger or Diane Sawyer, you might as well have TOURIST (or, alternately, ALSO-RAN) tattooed on your forehead. A big pile of beauty products on the table, bonanza as it might be for most people, telegraphs precisely the reason you're there. Without mystery in a New York restaurant, there is no power.

I did get over this, eventually, however. I came to the realization that Henry Kissinger and Diane Sawyer aren't wondering about me, mystery or no. The many years it took me to arrive at this realization doubtlessly indicate some sort of karmic debt being paid.

Behind just about every beauty product is a public relations person, and these people range dramatically in quality. It's a difficult job, in my estimation, and the good ones (and even some not so good) make enormous amounts of money, because doing it calling people on the phone and demanding, pleading, imploring them to put a particular item in the magazine; throwing big events designed to impress at times very imperious people; placating angry clients who make awful, uninspiring beauty products and can't understand why they aren't on the cover of *Vogue* would quickly send lesser souls right over the edge.

Marketing people are often also involved; either way, we eat our lunch and they hawk their wares. (I take the opportunity to sing my magazine's many virtues right back.)

Some people have to sing for their supper; the beauty editor thing with practically any product is to rub a little of whatever it is on the back of your hand, just by your thumb (where a makeup artist mixes colors), tilt your head in an evaluative slant, and then nod and "hmmm" your approval.

Perfume—the beauty equivalent of mystery meat—requires a decision about whether to spritz it on your naked wrist or onto a nearby napkin. The "industry professional" way to do it is to spritz it into the cap of the bottle, but I always forget and instead do an odd equation in my head involving how powerful the person is versus how likely it is that the perfume really stinks.

"So you see, we're really working within our core brand identity—taking our brand DNA and running with it," the person will say about a new fragrance that's exactly the same as the old one except there's now shimmer infused into it, or it's got patchouli added to it for depth, or they've made it "light" for summer.

The fragrance is always called the juice. "And the thing is, it's just a great juice," is what they always say, in a way that indicates a mild sense of surprise, as if the other "juices" they've pitched in the past weren't so wonderful, but this, this one is really something new.

Focus Groups and the Fragrance Industry

There is a single scent that everyone—everyone who's ever been in a focus group—loves at least in theory. It is a little flowery, a little fresh, a little fruity, and it "dries down" into something spicier and sexier. Practically every new fragrance smells this way, because this is what the people in the focus groups agree on. The cosmetics companies slap a different label on it, or put it in a different bottle, or attach a different celebrity to it, but it's the same. This is not to say the people working on each individual fragrance are simply copying one another; perfumers search far and wide for all sorts of exotic ingredients and ideas, mix them together in innovative ways—but the focus groups steer them inevitably to the flowery-fruity-fresh.

Big blockbuster fragrances, much like fancy face creams, are much more than simply what's in the bottle—it's what the ad says to you, what the bottle says to you, even what the color of the fragrance says to you, plus of course what it actually smells like that all add up to something you want to spritz on before your big night (or big board meeting, whatever). So buying a different flowery-fruity-fresh for every one of your moods still makes sense, in a way.

There are big fragrances that do smell different—Angel is one—that the industry refers to as "love it or hate it" fragrances. They don't make as much money as the flowery-fruity-fresh initially, but they hang around a lot longer—people are very loyal if they love a love-it-or-hate-it. Angel has been around for ten years. (I, incidentally, hate it on me: I remember trying it when it first came out, reeking immediately of pineapple and chocolate, and freaking out when I couldn't wash off the smell, so tenacious was the formula. But whenever I see Lisa Fernandez, the gorgeous fashion stylist, she smells fantastic; I ask what she's wearing, and she always says with a huge, triumphant smile on her face, "It's still Angel!")

It's the people who skip the focus groups altogether who produce the things I love. Lev Glazman, who runs the company Fresh with his wife, Alina, has produced a flowery-fruity-fresh only once, and it was after a bigger company bought his company and must've demanded that he use a focus group. He called me to ask about that particular one, and though I said I liked it (it was already packaged up and ready to go), I was unsurprised (and deeply saddened) when he noted, "The tests on this were through the roof."

Perfume: The Hardest Thing to Write About

I believe every one of my beauty editor colleagues is with me on this: Sit down one day and try to describe your favorite perfume in a few sentences. If you find it easy, describe two more—and the same word cannot be used more than once. You'll find yourself out of *sexy* and *floral* and *sweet* fairly fast. And what's sexy to one person is babyish to the next, what's light to others is overpowering to the people on the elevator. It's next to impossible to adequately describe what a perfume smells like. But we soldier on.

Most of Lev's creations, however, are the opposite. He was in Cape Cod, and some smell reminded him of being a teenager and camping out by the Red Sea—the sun, the sand, the Bedouins with their boiling cauldrons of exotic stew, the juniper berries . . . Watching him talk about different ingredients—how he mixed together this sugar scrub and then had the idea of throwing in this unexpected, weird element, the memory this one was a paean to—is unbelievably inspiring. A fragrance that Lev has worked on is like Le Cirque versus McDonald's: the inside of one person's mind versus something a stadium full of people can agree on.

The Stratum Corneum

Half of my free lunches are regular lunches, at restaurants; the other half are "events," where the cosmetics company invites all the beauty editors at once and does a big presentation after the lunch, the breakfast, the afternoon tea, whatever. The thing that the people throwing all the events don't understand, as I've mentioned, is that you still have to get the same amount of work done as the editor in the next cubicle, three-hour lunch or no.

(They also often forget to feed you. "Editors don't eat" is something I've heard over and over from PR executives. So they'll invite us for "lunch" at noon, offer a few scant hors d'oeuvres, and make their presentation for the next several hours. Not even the strictest Atkins adherent appreciates this; we emerge at 2:00 p.m. faint, resentful, and famished.)

The most common way to pay for your free lunch, regular or event based, actual food or pretend, is to listen to a lengthy

Creams

No matter what you pay for it, plain old moisturizer is no substitute for lost youth or, for that matter, a facelift. That said, moisturizer supercharged with antiaging ingredients does do something for most people, and even plain old moisturizer will make you look better—via the momentary effect of plumping up your skin so your wrinkles look less noticeable—temporarily. And I think the regular act of touching your skin in some caring, curative way probably helps as well.

There are things that they put in moisturizers that do work: alpha hydroxy acids, retinol, peptides, and vitamin C. The first three work by speeding up your skin's exfoliation: As you age, your skin exfoliates ever more slowly, so speeding it back up, in theory, is a powerful route back to a baby smooth complexion.

My personal favorite is some form of Retin-A (Renova, Tazorac, etc.), which really can make people look significantly younger. There was a woman named Fran at my first job in New York who must've been about forty at the time. She always looked a little funny, because she was in the art department and thus dressed very funkily—short shirts, lots of black, fingerless gloves, big clonking boots, very *Desperately Seeking Susan*—which was at odds with her not-fresh-out-of-college face. All of a sudden, Fran's face started matching her clothes; she no longer looked a little off-kilter; in fact, she looked hot. We all had to ask her why she looked so fabulous. "Retin-A!" she said triumphantly.

You have to be on Retin-A for about two months before you notice its amazing results, but they are *amazing*. My friend Jennifer and I both used it to temper our hideous acne until we both got pregnant (you have to quit Retin-A when you're pregnant, because it's related to Accutane, which causes birth defects). A month of two after we'd had the babies, one morning we happened to catch ourselves in the mirror of my upstairs bathroom, which, especially in winter, is flooded with a very harsh northern light. *Crestfallen* is a delicate term for the despair we shared at that moment. "We really need that Retin-A back," I said finally.

Once we did have it back (post-breast-feeding, etc.), we waited about six weeks and were thrillingly returned to our old, less lined selves.

discussion of the stratum corneum, otherwise known as the outer layer of your skin—never referred to as such by cosmetics companies, which think the fancy scientific name will bestow a glamorous sort of confusion that will make you think of them as knowledgeable experts.

At some point in most skin cream launches, the cosmetics company hauls out a French scientist—even if the company itself is not French, the scientist is invariably French, with a heavy accent. The combination of the long words and the accent serves again to create a sort of fog, wherein very simple things are made to sound complicated and mysterious, as in, "Zees moisturizer ees an eggzellent hydrator." Hydrator as in moisturizer. As in, "This automobile is an excellent car."

The French scientist then always brings out a diagram of the skin. I don't know why, but I find the words *follicle* and *sebum* to be extremely distasteful; each time I go through the stratum corneum discussion, I feel as if I'm having the details of menstruation diagrammed, or perhaps colon polyps.

The reason for the diagram is always the same: It's to show how hard it is to penetrate the skin. The endgame for all skin care and hair products is always penetration. "You see how zees cream actually penetrates zee skin," or, "Unlike other hair products, this conditioner/shampoo/hair color actually penetrates the hair shaft." *Penetrates the hair shaft.*

So there is always a second diagram/money shot, wherein little particles of the product are shown penetrating the stratum corneum. Everyone is happy when the nanospheres or the liposomes or the beta hydroxy acids finally penetrate the stratum corneum, because it means that lunch is over.

Acne Breakfast

There are, of course, far fouler things in store for the beauty editor than a lengthy discussion of the skin's barrier function. Over the course of my career, I have received not one but several invitations that read, in perfectly bold letters, "ACNE BREAKFAST," and I went only once. We sat at little desks with plates of eggs, smoked salmon, and strawberries and cream while the PR operative flashed some of the most horrific images I have ever seen (remember, I am a person who's had my share of acne) before us. No one ate much.

There are wrinkle symposia and rosacea lunches, but truly the worst for me was a teatime cellulite product launch. We sat, as always, at desks, this time with little plates of scones and clotted cream, tiny cupcakes, mini tarts, and jelly beans.

At the head of the "class" was a little stage, where the French scientists—in their white lab coats, scurrying around like the Oompah Loompah technicians that hustle Mike Teevee off to be stretched back out in *Charlie and the Chocolate Factory*—were in full swing with all sorts of ghastly diagrams. Suddenly, out of nowhere, they produced a woman—a bit on the heavy side, not terribly so—outfitted in a skimpy T-shirt and a pair of high-cut Dolphin running shorts.

This was a "small group" event, so there were perhaps about fifteen of us crowded in the small room; it was intimate. The woman in the running shorts stood facing us; on cue, she turned around to reveal . . . her cellulite. "THIS WOMAN HAS CELLULITE," boomed the announcer, pointing his pointer at the area and making circular motions. "YOU SEE IT HERE, AROUND THE UPPER THIGHS AND BUTTOCKS."

Acne

Everybody's plagued by it, and everybody thinks they're the only sufferer. It's by far the main reason people come into my office with a question. Men, women, old, young. Here's what I think actually helps:

- **A dermatologist.** If my parents had taken me to one in eighth or ninth grade, my entire high school and college life could have been drastically improved. It's worth the money. A dermatologist can get you Accutane (harsh, and you have to sign a form that says you'll get an abortion if you become pregnant, but everyone I know who's ever gone on it has the clearest skin ever and has spent the rest of their days so grateful to not have the horrible acne they once did). Dermatologists can also prescribe Retin-A, which works for lesser cases (I fit in this category). They can give you peels, laser treatments, and injections, all of which work.
- **A regimen.** I'm convinced that all the acne-guru products work to the degree they do because people get inspired and they actually cleanse and tone (though I think toner's useless) and treat their acne every day. The problem is, you have to *keep* doing it, every day, and once most people's skin clears up, they breathe a sigh of relief and think, Ah, now I can quit! And a week later they're breaking out again, and they run out and buy a new regimen.
- **Compliance.** I've just said this, but I mean it. Whatever you do, keep doing it, forever, long after your skin's clear. You don't cure acne; you just vigilantly, constantly, remove the bacteria that cause it. For that reason, pick a regimen with the fewest steps possible, so you're more likely to stick with it. Seventeen steps every night is a sure route to failure, not to mention wild expenditure.

They rolled out a sonogram machine to document the cellulite (in case we were having trouble seeing it): One "scientist" rubbed gel on the back of the woman's upper thigh; another approached with the unbelievably phallic, giant dildo sonogram sensor and moved it tentatively up and down across her skin. Up on the screen, the "results" of the sonogram mapped—in wavy, blubbery lines—the grave extent of the cellulite. "SO YOU SEE, THIS WOMAN REALLY HAS A PROBLEM."

Another scientist gingerly applied the anticellulite lotion—the way a shy man might struggle though a lap dance at a bachelor party. The woman turned back to face us again, so they could map the cellulite on her outer thigh. We struggled to appear attentive while avoiding the poor woman's eyes. "PROBLEMS HERE, TOO, YOU SEE," continued the an-

Cellulite

Never, ever, have I seen something that totally gets rid of cellulite. Even cosmetics companies don't really claim this. The *appearance* is another thing, but to get *rid* of it, I'm sorry, losing weight is the only viable strategy. If you rub a cream—any cream—faithfully on your thighs for six weeks, you'll think you see a difference. If you pay someone to rub in that cream for you, you'll see an even bigger difference.

Important Codicil: Self-tanner is right up there with well-cut black pants in terms of *disguising* cellulite. It can make bathing suit shopping downright enjoyable.

nouncer. At the end (it lasted about two hours), we got gift bags containing the anticellulite lotion—and a whole big bunch of candy.

Does It Work?

The other big word in skin care is *active*. The products are always "very active" or "full of actives," and the companies are always striving to demonstrate these properties. There was an oddly un-French scientist who ran the research department of an enormous American company and on a number of occasions (for several different creams for several different brands) used a small crystal tied to a string to show the "high levels of actives" in the cream. He suspended the crystal over the open jar of cream and explained how the molecules in the cream would somehow excite the crystal (or perhaps the air around it?). "You see how I'm not moving my hand at all," he said, shaking his hand vigorously to make the crystal go around and around in a circular pattern. "And you see how the crystal is starting to make movements all on its own?"

I think of my father at these moments. His head would just explode.

The way they demonstrate a product's effectiveness is always the same (excepting innovations like the cellulite sonogram): with a graph detailing the percentage of the focus-group women who tried the product and saw a noticeable difference in their skin or who said they intended to purchase it once it was available. The percentages are always astounding, in the eighties and nineties. This only gives credence to my theory that everyone loves a beauty product and if you bottled pond scum (plant extracts and a rare Appalachian algae complex), people would line up for it.

The Emperor's New Clothes

Once I received a tube of eyelash balm—think about this for a minute—to condition your lashes and treat any brittle ones. ("I love her, she's just so beautiful, if only her eyelashes weren't so brittle and dull!") Strangely, a few days later I went to lunch to hear about a new, clear eye shadow. "It's for that customer who really likes a natural look," the publicist explained earnestly. I opened up the little pot of it and touched it. It looked sort of like lip balm, except more matte. "So it's shiny?" I said. "It's about a texture?"

"Well, the texture is very subtle, which is what's so nice about it," the woman continued. "It's just so easy, and so natural, and it's almost impossible to make a mistake!"

The thing about a product that does nothing is it actually delights people. One co-worker was in my office at least twice a day, all over that clear, textureless eye shadow: "Can you see it? Can you tell I'm wearing it? Do I look any different?" Even though the answer was always an emphatic "No!" he kept coming back for it. He even sampled the eyelash balm.

My cousin Sara (of cancer research fame) and I once locked ourselves in the bathroom for hours to put highlights in our hair. We sat on the side of the tub in those awful plastic caps, combing the bleach onto the tiniest strands of hair, leaving it on for the least amount of time possible. When we finally emerged, we were thrilled to look precisely the same as we had when we went in. "No one's going to be able to tell!" pronounced my cousin, triumphant. Secret—even very secret—transformation is a powerful thing.

Photo Shoot

A common gambit for makeup events is to have a famous (or relatively famous) photographer take a picture of each editor with all the makeup on. Thus I have a gallery of large (eleven-by-eighteen and up), uniformly alarming (under the best of conditions I do not photograph well) portraits of myself. Who, besides I guess a top model, needs a big fat picture of themselves? A big fat picture of you and some other people, or in a particular place, might have some meaning, but just a great big portrait? You'd need a great deal of regard and affection for yourself to want to look at yourself on the mantelpiece every day.

The best of these "shoots" was for a makeup company whose creative director was also a photographer. I arrived at the glamorous Industria studio at 8:30 in the morning, suspecting nothing. A makeup artist piled makeup on me; I was a little hung over. I sat there calculating how long it was going to take me to get all the eye shadow off in the cab on the way to the office. I was led into a second room—a cavernous studio complete with billowing white curtains and huge hot photo lights, Foreigner blasting on the stereo. "Oh no," I said. "I'm really not photogenic—no, thank you!"

But of course they insisted: The famous photographer would be taking my picture! The famous photographer was a wiry, rock-star-looking character, all tight pants, unbuttoned-to-there blousy-type shirt, a big seventies shag, boots. If you needed a "hot fashion photographer" from Central Casting, this is the guy they'd send you.

"Hey, babe!" he yelled, jumping into place in time with the music. *Girl I'm HOT-BLOODED, check it and see . . .* There was no turning back.

"Stand right there, yeah, YEEEAH, oh yeah, GORGEOUS, honey!" Again with the Central Casting, this time with the dialogue. Yeah, I'm *HOT-BLOODED* . . . I knew the charade would all come to an end when he had a look at the Polaroids (photographers always take a few Polaroids before they shoot actual film, so they can tell if their lighting's right and if the pictures are good).

He took one look at the Polaroids and suggested a wind machine. If you didn't know better, you might think, A wind machine! So glamorous! But the sad reality is that a wind machine is what they use when they need something—anything—to help make a picture attractive. Perhaps all the flying hair takes your mind off the person's face. I swallowed my pride and tried to appear excited over the fact that a wind machine was necessary.

He flipped on the wind machine and turned up the music even louder. "Yeah! ALL RIIIIGHT!" He squirmed in his tiny jeans, his shag flipping around excitedly as he snap-snap-snapped. Very Duran Duran. The wind machine, alas, was a little dusty; I'm allergic to just about everything that moves, particularly dust, and the machine blew it all directly into my eyes.

I got a fever of 103 . . . Tears started streaming down my face as if I'd just been left at the altar. I could feel my eyes going the bright swelling red that they do in these situations. The tears were mixing with the not-insignificant amount of eye

Looking Good in Pictures

- The most flattering light is what photographers call "full shade": You're in the shade, but it's sunny outside. A close second is an overcast day.
- Look at the camera and (in general) smile. A calculated nonsmile can look contrived and I'm-too-sexy-for-my-shirt. Models and celebs spend hours in front of the mirror (or, more effectively, with a Polaroid) figuring out the best smile, angle, etc. I've never done this, but I don't know why I haven't, since I'm one of the most unphotogenic people alive; it's a fifteen-minute investment (albeit a self-absorbed one you wouldn't want to broadcast at your next cocktail party, but whatever) that'll pay off the rest of your life.
- Natural makeup is the only way to go, period. Think Bobbi Brown and never stray. Think of the glam-y, makeup-y Lauren Hutton shoots where she either looked significantly older, or like a prostitute, or, in the worst case, like an old prostitute. In the natural-makeup Barneys Steven Meisel ones, she's her unbelievably breathtaking self.
- Blue is a very flattering (clothing) color on most people. This is especially important if you're going on TV; film can overamplify many colors into the lurid range very easily.
- Black-and-white film is generally more forgiving.
- You can wear a great deal more makeup if you're being photographed in black and white.
- If it's a portrait sort of situation, get the photographer to take as many shots as humanly possible.

makeup they'd applied and doubtlessly streaking down in greasy, bruise-colored rivulets; the wildly churning hair kept catching in the mixture and sticking to my cheeks.

"YOU LOOK SO HOT!" he just kept going, pretending everything was completely normal. "Yeah, babe, give me a smile! SO HOT! UH-HUH! One more smile!"

I received the photograph in the mail several weeks later, complete with the makeup they'd used to "create the look." It was a lesson for me in the true powers of retouching: not a tear on my face, not the slightest puffiness around the eyes. It did not look terribly like me, however (there was a decided Stepford quality), except for the fact that it was not a pretty picture, which, for me, is par for the course.

Top Experts

Like French scientists at skin cream launches, hairstylists are usually in evidence at hair events, as are makeup artists at makeup events. These people have a good deal more credibility, in general, than the French scientists. They work with hair or makeup all day, with real people—as opposed to focus groups and target markets and cosmetic laboratories. Some have their own lines, and some are paid by companies to represent their products. The only problem occurs when the companies hire people pretending to be something they're not.

There's a tragic situation wherein a cosmetics company will pay a makeup artist or hairstylist who hasn't been to the fashion shows to report to us beauty editors on the "trends" from the "shows." Thousands of makeup artists *do* attend the fashion shows, creating the makeup for them, but this man or woman would not be among them. Most beauty editors also attend the shows; we work for *fashion* magazines, after all. Nonetheless, we sit through lengthy lunches, listening to blustery postulates about what might or might not be in style.

"What we're seeing now is a return to innocence," the uninformed makeup artist will venture with the air of an embedded CNN correspondent. "Think pink, girls! Pink Twinkler Eye Quad Palette! Blend it with the Cheeky Pink blush duo!" Their commentary tends to come straight off the press release: "What we're seeing is major drama, girls! Be a drama queen!" At one event, we received a lecture, museum-docent style, on various *furniture* trends throughout the ages, which the hired makeup artist (cum art historian) had been charged with connecting—however tangentially—to the company's new makeup shades.

Graft

You leave your lunch or your event with a gift bag; in it are the products and, often, a gift. You get so much free stuff as a beauty editor that you quickly become ungrateful and jaded. And you get so much that you also quickly become unbiased; the gifts cease to have much meaning, especially because most of them are thought up by clever marketers to in some way reflect the theme of whatever they're sending. I have so many plastic pails and shovels (goes with sunscreen!), I literally couldn't count them if I tried; ditto flip-flops (nail polish) and terrycloth robes (any spa-themed item). I've been sent thong underwear on at least ten separate occasions (would you send someone you didn't know a thong? even if you were pushing hair removal cream?), enough candy and cookies to feed a significant portion of the world's population (never send people sweets; for a single moment they love you, and then they spend the rest of the day cursing you), and cameras galore (you use your EYES to look through a camera, so they often accompany new collections of eye makeup).

Then there are the total non sequiturs: Once, in a cab back from a new makeup launch, I opened up the bag to see what the gift was. There were the various products, along with a long thin tube, like one that might contain a small poster. I opened it and out fell a purple beret, not unlike the one famously worn by Monica Lewinsky. As I puzzled over the connection, a Chipmunk-like voice chirped from the tube: "She wore a RASPBERRY beret, the kind you find . . ." I slammed the top back on and rifled through the makeup again, trying to understand. I opened the tube afresh, in disbelief (I'm sure the cab driver was confused as well), and the Chipmunk voice began again. Back in the office, when I read the press release, I noted that a raspberry-shaded lipstick had been highlighted.

I have a special drawer in my office full of such gifts—the Botox-emblazoned coffee mug, a giant ceramic nose glued to a small pedestal, a pen that looks like a syringe (complete with red "blood" sloshing around inside of it), mini camouflage-printed underwear stuffed with potpourri. Random. Puzzling.

Some of the gifts, though, are fantastic. Kiehl's was famous at one time for giving enormous, over-the-top Christmas gifts (entire Prada outfits, Cartier watches, that sort of thing). They never advertised in magazines, and people assumed they just bought their way in with the Christmas presents. But as anyone who's ever been in a Kiehl's store knows, you don't need to bribe someone to get them to say how great the products are.

The first time I heard of Kiehl's was before I was a beauty editor, and my friend and I were immediately glamorized. It was literally blizzarding in New York, everything was shut down, but we had to have it. We walked—through the driving snow—all the way to Barneys to get it, but they were out of stock. So we went back into the whirling maelstrom and proceeded all the way across town to the Kiehl's store. We got there, barely able to speak, ice hanging from our eyebrows, and thawed slowly in the bewildering entryway—all sorts of seemingly unrelated paraphernalia and printed tracts about aviation and downhill skiing—slowly becoming aware of the row upon satisfyingly straightforward row of products we were dying to rip from the shelves. We spent hundreds of dollars, which we were in no position to do at the time; loaded down with our loot—including the many generously sized free samples the friendly salespeople gave us—we trudged back through the even heavier snow, happier than happy.

The thing I've learned from all the gifts is that small-time bribery doesn't work. It fails to inspire even the tiniest bit of friendly feeling and just leaves the recipient clawing ungracefully for more. As anyone who's bought anything at a cosmetics counter in the past twenty years finds when they unwrap the vinyl makeup bag with the discontinued lipstick sample and the fuchsia eye shadow inside, something that's free that's not quite what you'd have picked for yourself is not quite . . . satisfying. You keep it around—because you should use it! after all, it was *free!*—and it collects dust pitifully. My basement is clogged with soapdishes made to look like bathtubs, weird miniature mailboxes, plastic fruit, handbags that have it all wrong. . . . I keep them, thinking there must eventually be some use for them, and eventually I give them to charity, at last endowing my lame defeat with some modicum of dignity.

And then the next odd knicknack/gift/bribe crosses my desk and I snap it up like a chimpanzee snatching at a morsel of banana. And the cycle begins anew. . . .

What does work, on the other hand, is saying "Thank you." I know I sound like someone's grandmother, but I can remember just about everything I ever received in the form of a thank-you and exactly whom I received it from, whether it was flowers, or a note, or what. There's something about knowing that someone saw something you did, and appreciated it, that's innately satisfying and gives you a warm, fuzzy feeling about the person that's hard to erase. If you want people to love you, send them thank-you notes instead of love letters.

Your other option is to take out an ad. Taking out lots of ads in a women's fashion magazine is a much surer thing than sending chocolates, or even Prada handbags, if it's the attention of the beauty editor you're trying to get.

The thing to remember, though, before you reject all beauty editor advice as biased, bribery-induced pap, is that just about every beauty line has some great items and some awful ones. I for one (and most of my compatriots) simply don't write about the awful ones. We also can't resist a great beauty product; gifts, ads or no, the great stuff (Kiehl's, etc.) is always going to make it in.

The Donald

You wouldn't think of Donald Trump as a big beauty operative, but perhaps because of the whole model thing, our worlds kept colliding. The first was at the U.S. Open, which Kiehl's used to invite us to every year. Kiehl's used to be owned by a very rich, eccentric, and generous couple, who among other stunning favors (see "Graft") sent a group of us to the men's final every year, always in heart-stoppingly good seats. This particular year we were seated with the Donald in his box. He was there with Marla, she in white short-shorts, he in an ill-fitting red blazer that looked hot (it was about eighty-nine degrees and very sunny).

His young son slid into the seat on the end. "Oh no, son, you're going to have to move," blared the Donald, waving his arms impatiently. "You gotta move! I have to sit there, because that's where all the cameras are going to be! They need to see me!" He settled in and started ordering food, furiously: hot dogs, fries, candy bars, drinks. He had a bite or so of a hot dog and began handing out the rest to everyone. The kids took a few items, Marla naturally demurred; he offered some to us, then to the people below him. He spotted Georgette Mosbacher a few rows down. "Georgette!" he screamed. "Georgette, you want some chocolate? Some candy bars?" She waved happily, uncomprehending, and he sent down several cardboard boxes of the hot, melting, unnaturally bright food.

It was hot; the sun was going down, right in our eyes. You could see the sweat in balls on the top of his head, beneath his reddish hair. There were visors on each person's seat that read INFINITY or LEXUS or something, so we all put them on to stop squinting so we could actually see the game. Marla handed him one as he sat there, squinting. (I realized that day something about trophy/gold digger/whatever-you-want-to-call-it wives: They are, practically by definition, very nice, tolerant people. Because taking care of—placating—Donald Trump and his ilk requires SuperMom powers beyond those of most minivan-wielding, nose-wiping, boo-boo-kissing saints.)

"MARLA, ARE YOU CRAZY?" he yelled (yes, there is a bit of Owen Meany about Donald Trump), wagging the visor close to her face. "If I put this visor on, the cameras are going to catch it. It's like I'm endorsing it, and half the people in America are going to go buy a Lexus!" He dispatched a bodyguard to his car to get him a visor emblazoned with TRUMP PARC or some such.

Then his daughter, Ivanka—who had not yet turned glamorous and was simply this beautiful little girl just back from summer camp, tanned, in Levi's jeans and a pair of Birkenstocks, maybe twelve—was talking to some very cute boys, her age, about the camp from which they'd apparently all just returned. "IVANKA," he said over their voices. "*IVANKA!* DO YOU ACTUALLY KNOW THESE PEOPLE, OR ARE THEY JUST FANS?"

Then there was the time Trump invited all the beauty editors down to see his new spa at Mar-a-Lago in Palm Beach—just for the day. He flew us down on his private plane, which was not your usual kind of private plane, but a full-on, 747 kind of plane that would normally have rows and rows of seats but instead had sofas and king-size beds and bathrooms with gold-plated faucets. "You're perfectly safe, girls," he kept telling us. "I have the best pilot money can buy." This did make me feel safe, actually; I am terrified of flying, but I imagined him offering United's best pilot double his salary, and my heart rate immediately went down several notches.

"If this plane goes down, you know," he said, sending my heart rate back up, "they're not going to be looking for you, and they're not even going to be looking for me!" He smiled and pointed. "They're going to be looking for that Renoir over there. It's worth three million dollars!"

Most of the way down, he detailed how much money he'd suckered people out of on various real estate deals, punctuated with admonishments not to forget about the Renoir. Then he got bored and wanted to show someone the cockpit; as the Donald is unsurprisingly label conscious, the beauty editor of *Vogue* and I *(Elle)* were chosen to go. He let us sit in the jump seat right behind the two pilots, un-seat-belted in, as the plane first slowed, then began to dip, ever more steeply, banking all the way down to Palm Beach Airport as we first landed and then taxied down the runway. It was glorious. Being able to see what the pilot was doing (I might have felt differently had there been fog or rain or something, but it was crystal-clear) made everything all right. More than all right: I've never enjoyed a plane ride quite as much as that one.

Now that the Donald has a fragrance (Trump, distributed by Estée Lauder and wildly successful), our worlds again recently collided. For the launch, the beauty editors were all brought into The Boardroom. We got him to say, "You're fired!" a couple of times, and we even got to meet the hard-charging Carolyn. The best part was going down in the elevator afterward, exiting the building, and hailing a cab, exactly the way the hapless losers do it on TV. If they'd packaged up our press materials in a roll-away suitcase instead of a bag, the picture would have been complete.

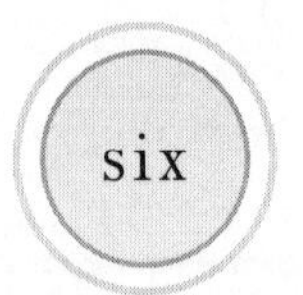

The Night No One Recognized Me

The beauty closet is a beautiful thing, but it pales in comparison with the fashion closet. While the things in the beauty closet don't have to be sent back to their manufacturers, the things in the fashion closet do. But you can borrow them if you can fit in them, if you're friends with the fashion editors.

The beauty editor job involves many fancy but not exactly chic parties, usually black tie, usually held in large hotel ballrooms. If your fashion-closet-controlling coworkers like you, they take pity on you and loan you free clothes (and shoes and bags) for the evening. It's very Cinderella, especially when combined with getting your hair, nails, and makeup done for free. I always kept the pretty-dress machine well oiled with a constant flow of beauty products from my office into the fashion department. Though I am not the size of a model, I'm the size a model *would* be, except she's much taller. So the model's dress still fits, though it's a bit longer on me, which, if you think about it, is all well and good.

About a month into my new job at *Elle*, I got my first black-tie invitation. "What should I wear?" I asked my boss.

"Come on," she said, "let's go to the fashion closet. They already called in something for me." She marched me down the hall to the fashion editor (we'll call her Fashionista), whose innate scariness (all fashion editors are commanding, disdainful, cruel) was enhanced by the fact that she happened to be a movie star's daughter and at times resembled the sinister, hyperventilating characters her father was famous for in disturbing ways. She had fired the entire fashion department on more than one occasion, and she could not have been more terrifying.

"We have that black tie; got anything?" my boss kindly asked for me.

After returning with my boss's preordered, wildly gorgeous ball gown, Fashionista regarded me. "What do you want?"

"Uh, oh, anything, you know," I managed. She went back and rummaged for a moment, then returned, grudgingly, with the most beautiful silver slip dress you can imagine from Ghost. "I need it back in three days," she said slowly, breathing, her eyes boring into me. "If—you—do—anything—to—it, I—will—kill—you."

The night of the event, I went to get my hair done at a fancy salon. It looked great, swoopy, swirly, big-night-out-y. When it was done, they wanted to do my makeup. In fact, the makeup artist was already there, ready to go, dying to do it. In my inexperience, I didn't feel I could say no, despite the fact that even that early on, I knew the effects of "makeovers" were rarely positive things for me.

There's a picture of me at fourteen, in full high school dance attire, posing seductively after a visit to the Merle Norman store at the mall with my friend: I look like a teenage runaway in the parking lot of a truck stop. Heavy eyeliner, a rainbow with subtle gradations of eye shadow that fans to my brow bone, visible lip liner, great clownlike splotches of blush, and contouring powder, all of it. We've all learned it at one makeup counter or another: Free makeovers are rarely what they're cracked up to be. And subtlety is rarely the issue.

This free makeover involved actual *body* makeup (I thought, Maybe this is what people do when they go to black ties), along with lots and lots of solid-silver eye shadow. Pancake-y base; layers of thick concealer and powder; amazing amounts of blush to define not just my cheekbones but also my jawline, plus that midcheek area where you're supposed to have hollows; eyeliner and more eyeliner and then eyeliner on top of that; mascara like the goopiest, drippiest black-tar soup; darkish mauve lipstick. The body makeup was thick and tan ("This'll make the silver on the dress stand out," the makeup artist murmured approvingly*) and somehow both stain-y and cakey.

***Silver really plays up a tan.** Even more than white.

As I rose to leave, she whipped out a big brush covered with bronzing powder, which she shook all over me. "Now it won't budge," she said, her voice filled with satisfaction.

My most powerful stress reduction technique is denial, and it works (why look at your watch when you know you're already late and you're stuck in the most hideous traffic jam ever encountered? Read *US Weekly* and add a few years to your life while you're at it). So I didn't even really look at myself in the mirror when the maquillage was complete—what could I have done about it at that point? I got into the cab and off to my event.

Over the Top?

Too much makeup, as this fiasco demonstrates, can really be a bummer, but being too dressed up is nothing to worry about, ever. You just look more glamorous, interesting, and adventurous than everyone else. I had a friend who wore thick silk bias-cut slips all day on the weekends, for the grungiest situations. Even taking out the garbage, she looked like some heiress from the twenties about to have her next sip of champagne.

It was horrifying to be all dressed up and strangely naked at the same time, smiling at people who all seemed to know one another and not me. At last I caught sight of my friend (another beauty editor) and her husband; we'd been sharing a summer house. I rushed over to greet them—and they smiled at me politely, uncomprehendingly. I finally had to say, "It's me . . . Jean? Jean Godfrey-June?"

"Wow, that's some amazing makeup they put on you," the husband finally managed.

Four hours later, somewhat humiliated yet exhilarated at having survived my big night, I returned home, still caked with makeup. "How was it?" Gary asked. My penchant for drama did not waver: I marched to the bathroom, got out an enormous, deeply glamorous pump bottle of Princess Marcella Borghese makeup remover, and hurled myself into a kitchen chair, thumping the bottle down directly in front of me. I leaned heavily on the pump mechanism, hoping to squirt a bit into some Kleenex. Instead a huge slosh of it shot out like paint from a paintball gun, dead center into the middle of the gorgeous, solid silver Ghost dress.

Known, Proven, True

This rule is controversial among beauty editors, but I stand by it: If you're putting on makeup for a big night out, focus on your eyes or your lips, but not both. Go for gorgeous red lipstick but forgo the bronzed shimmer power. Go for the bronzed shimmer powder and do some nude, shiny lip gloss. If you wear it all together, the effect is more lady-of-the-night (or man-dressed-as-lady-of-the-night).

I spent the next three days practically anaphylactic with fear and dread, knowing I'd be fired if I couldn't get the dress clean, visiting and revisiting the unsympathetic (aren't they all) dry cleaners. Miraculously, on the third try, the fabulous silver dress emerged from its wrapper—to the skeptical clucks of the dry-cleaning clerk—spotless. It was the greatest day of my life, and I remained at my post at *Elle.*

Beyond the never-let-them-have-their-way-with-you-again lesson I learned that night, the general Cinderella feeling of the black tie gave way to its true nature: Dressed up or not, everyone's working. They're connecting, they're networking, they're supporting, they're whispering, they're laughing—and besides the fabulous outfits, you might as well be on the convention floor in AnyHotel, USA.

Like some Zen koan, I think, the point of getting dressed up is, in fact, the getting dressed up. It's all about the process, right?

Perhaps it's the haze of alcohol and marijuana that punctuated most of these evenings, but I remember the getting ready part of the high school dance experience much more vividly

Eyeliner

I think eyeliner is a thousand times sexier than eye shadow. For those (like me) who can't put it on, get a dark eye shadow powder, lick the end of an eyeliner brush, tap it into the powder, and then place it, brush length by brush length, along your lash line, starting where you want the darkest spot to be (usually the outer edges). Keep going till it looks right. If it's too much and you hate it, wet a Q-tip (foully, I just again lick the end of it, but whatever) and erase away. Jeanine Lobell (of Stila) taught me this trick, and her brush and eye shadow are truly genius.

Even better, a number of companies (including the brilliant Stila) have now come out with gel eyeliner, which is more like a wax or pomade; applied the same way, with the same flat brush, you get the same look without the tendency of the shadow to sprinkle across your cheekbones like fairy dust, sprinkles that later erupt into enormous streaks of black or dark brown if you happen to brush your hand across them.

than the actual dance itself. I remember the kohl eye pencil from Lancôme that my friend was willing to share with us if we all agreed to get ready at her house, the hot curler set we fried our hair with in her mom's glamorous 1970s–1980s master bath, with its reflective wallpaper and the pore-magnifying makeup mirror. The waxy-flavored lip gloss the fried curls would stick to, the perfume (one of us had Chloé, another Cinnabar, and other Lauren; whichever house we were at, that's what we wore).

When I was working at the ad agency in Cincinnati, I was very excited to go to my first big work Christmas party. The production company we worked with was throwing it; they were wildly hip in my estimation—we'd spend hours in the

Workout Makeover

I went to a party for a top, top makeup artist. I was late; I had squeezed in a yoga class before and was literally still sweating. As I've mentioned, I'm big into denial as a coping strategy. If I'm stuck in traffic, I don't look at my watch. If I'm still dripping with sweat from yoga as I'm walking into an elegant party—well, I pretend I'm not. I put on some lip gloss, spritzed a little perfume, and walked in.

"WHO DID YOUR MAKEUP?" demanded the top, top, international makeup artist.

"Your makeup looks so pretty!" exclaimed the president of the makeup company throwing the party.

"Did you have your makeup done?" queried a fellow beauty editor.

A few minutes later, another beauty editor appeared, even later than I, looking unusually stunning. "You look incredible!" I said.

"Oh God, I'm so late—I came straight from the gym! I'm still sweating," she whispered, "and I haven't even put on makeup! Can you tell?"

editing room working on commercials, living it up on shots of Jolt! (the cola with all the sugar and twice the caffeine). I knew the party was going to be unbelievably sophisticated, like something I'd never seen.

There was no fashion to be had in Cincinnati, so I drove the five hours (one way) to the mall in Cleveland, Ohio, that I believed to be the epicenter of all that was glamorous, owing to the two stupendously fashionable stores within it—Ann Taylor and Laura Ashley. I bought (with the two cents I had at that point) a purple satin shirt at Ann Taylor, got back in my car, and drove right back to Cincinnati, triumphant. The next day—very craftily, I thought—I arrived in a department store precisely at five and chose a makeup counter where they were featuring lots of watery-looking purples and blues on their collateral materials. The woman there gave me the full treatment, purple eye shadow, glossy lilac lips, all of it. Much to her chagrin, I bought nothing: "Um, I need to think about everything. . . ." Hopefully this was not the straw that broke the camel's back, leaving her forever jaded and embittered as to the inner workings of the human heart, but perhaps it was.

I left the counter at 5:30, fully satisfied and brimming with confidence. And though I can remember the exact shades of eye shadow I had on, I now couldn't tell you even a smidgen of what went on at the party. Or what it looked like. Or who was there. All I do know is that I had a good time—I came prepared.

The Fifis

I was unprepared for the beauty editor's most important black tie: The fragrance industry's annual awards are called, without the slightest touch of irony or embarrassment, the Fifi Awards. For a long time they were run by a tiny, shrill, and very powerful woman—we'll call her Marionette—who ran the Fragrance Foundation, which puts on the Fifis. There are Fifi ceremonies all over the world; Marionette attended all of them.

At our own, lengthy American Fifi ceremony, "celeb" presenters like Tova Borgnine and Priscilla Presley would unveil awards to tearful, loquacious winners, everyone taking their cues from the Oscars: "And the winner in the Men's Mass Market Scented-Lotion Products category is . . ."

"I just want to thank . . . my mom, God, and the whole marketing and sales team, Bobby, Janie, Stephanie . . ."

Since Marionette enjoyed international travel, we were always treated to a slide show where Marionette, Zelig-like, appeared in each photograph, at a different Fifi ceremony across the globe. "In March it was Paris . . . in April, on to Berlin!"

The Fifis were at Lincoln Center; they started at 6:30, and such was the power of tiny Marionette that she actually had the doors of Alice Tully Hall physically shut and locked at 6:31 to discourage latecomers. And you can't miss the Fifis if you're in the beauty industry. You might as well pack up and go home.

This particular year, the people at Armani (who make beautiful fragrances) invited me to the Fifis. Sometimes, if the beauty people who invite you are part of a fashion company (or, as in most cases, own the license to the fashion designer's name), they'll offer to lend you a dress by that designer for the night. This sounds good, but the choices can be limited.

Perfume

If you love it, wear it—that's pretty much all there is to perfume. Perfume can be the most charming thing in the world and it can be the most offensive, and it depends on who you are.

While I think the whole "layering" concept is a crock and an ill-disguised bid to get you to spend more money, I love the idea of *mixing* different fragrances, a practice that ends up costing just as much. This scented cream, plus this scented oil, plus this perfume . . . what's not to like?

They invited me to wear Armani, so they sent me down to a showroom, where I was offered a choice of two dresses. I was feeling grotesque that day, and after squeezing, sausagelike, into a pale stretch silk number that made me look, at best, like an asymmetrical mealybug (Sharon Stone looked much better in it when she wore it), I decided not to try on the other one and just take it. It was a long flowing skirt and a little beaded top; how bad could it be?

Several weeks later, the night of the Fifis had come, and I was late: I'd had my hair done at a glamorous salon in the Chelsea Hotel, but it had taken about six hours. I rushed home, did a five-second makeup job (I had learned my lesson about makeup artists by then), threw on the gorgeous beaded top and skirt—and noted that the top was completely see-through. Nor would any sort of undergarment that I had work at all. Nor had the pashmina craze hit, nor would a sweater work. And I literally had fifteen minutes to make it all the way uptown and into my seat for the Fifis.

It wasn't that sort of mysterious, feminine sort of see-through; it was "Have you ever wondered precisely what my breasts look like?" see-through, but there was nothing for it.

Once again with the denial: It's going to be dark, I reasoned. And how many people will really see me, anyway? I'd cross my arms and hope for the best.

Somehow I made it uptown by 6:31 and slid gratefully into my seat, breathing an enormous sigh of relief that I'd made it. The lights were already down, and I knew I had a good four hours of Fifi watching before I'd again have to think about the fact that I was half-naked.

"And the winner is . . . Jean Godfrey-June from *Elle!*" boomed the announcer on the stage. I hadn't realized there was

Evening Makeup

- The only thing an evening bag needs to be able to fit is a cell phone. If the cell phone fits, you should also have room for lipstick or lip gloss and concealer (the last only if there's some egregious spot with the potential to become uncovered during the course of the evening). Perfume maybe. Take along anything more than that, and you're going to feel ugly instead of pretty. Plus, full maquillage routines in public bathrooms are a Brechtian, pointless horror.
- Your skin doesn't really need powder at night. The idea is to glow, not to look professional.
- Use body makeup only if you are very skilled at the trapeze and/or the elaborate craft of mime.

a Fifi media award, but there was, and I had won it. And the packed Alice Tully Hall was waiting for me to come up and accept it.

I had to first walk down the enormous main aisle with a spotlight trained on me, then take the stage. I leaned into the podium as best I could to obscure my essentially naked breasts. "Um, thank you," I blurted boorishly. "This is an incredible honor." And I raced off the stage. Afterward, still under bright lights, I had to pose for pictures, the thin crystal Fifi the only thing to hide behind.

All night, well-wishers came up to congratulate me, trying hard not to look lower than my neck and wincing visibly at my lame attempts to joke about it. Thankfully, since the theme of the Fifis that year was "Stop and Smell the Memories—of Tomorrow!," the dinner (it began at 11:00 p.m., when the awards themselves were over) was decorated in a rudimentary sort of *Star Wars* aesthetic involving lots of black lights and star-shaped cutouts, so you could barely see anything, and somehow I survived.

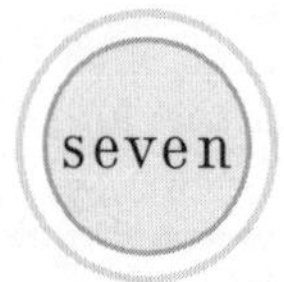

Queen at Last: How I Clawed My Way to the Top

However crazy the events and the black ties, the real challenge once I got to *Elle*—as it is for any beauty editor, at any magazine—was in the office. It was a crazy place. All fashion magazines are crazy places; the subjective nature of fashion and beauty means that success and failure are measured in similarly arbitrary ways. Your magazine can be selling well, both to readers and advertisers, and you can still get fired, simply because enough people decide that you're tired, or over, or whatever. Something gorgeous to one higher-up is hideous and embarrassing to the next. Everybody wants to sit in the front row, everybody's got to make a dramatic pronouncement, everybody wants that fabulous bag. . . . Fashion is rough, no matter what the context.

In ninth grade, my friend Julia and I got Christmastime jobs at Contempo Casuals in the mall. All the salesgirls at Contempo Casuals were superhot California-girl nineteen-year-olds in tailored pants and high-heeled boots; at Christmas, however, they were desperate for help, and standards had to be lowered. "Um, you know you're just working here for, like, just the Christmas rush?" said the manager, flicking back her long blond hair with the perfectly sharpened pencil in her manicured hand. "Like after Christmas we won't need you anymore? O-kee? . . . Great!"

Julia got the more glamorous position: She was actually out in front, greeting customers with the "Omigod! That skirt is SO CUTE!" pickup lines they taught us in the training and making real-life sales. I was just the add-on girl behind the counter. "You might want these earrings—they're SO CUTE with that angora sweater! There was a guy in here yesterday that got the sweater, the earrings, these bracelets, and the suede pants all together for his girlfriend! Like, a whole outfit?" I also helped wrap up everything we talked the poor people into.

I was the lowest of the low, but it was Julia they made miserable. "Um, honey?" one of the older salesgirls would say, descending upon her. "That outfit you are wearing is, um, not cute." On one occasion, they made her go all the way home (on her moped, in the rain) and change, despite the fact that we were in a store full of clothes. These incidents naturally occurred on lower-traffic days, with fewer customers to fight over for commissions.

My outfits were at least as not cute, but the salesgirls were always nice to me and never sent me home. Nobody wanted to do the job I was doing, so they loved me.

Fashion magazines provide a similar environment for the beauty editor: Beauty's just not as glamorous or interesting as fashion. And it brings in lots of money, so they leave you alone.

Beyond that, like everyone else on earth, the individual fashion people hanker after this skin cream or that lip gloss, so at the end of the day, most of them are nice to you.

This dynamic was firmly in place at *Elle,* where the politics swirled even more wildly than usual, thanks to the uneasy détente between the French, who ran half the magazine, and the Americans, who ran the other.

At one end of the building, the stunning corner office belonged to the man I'll call the Playboy, the French creative director/head photographer. To his left was the fashion department, to his right was the art department. The Playboy was short, jovial, and even charming, fiftyish with curly hair and a golden tan, almost always in white jeans and a gray T-shirt. He was aggressively heterosexual enough that the scarves he wore every day and the red leather Fendi bag he carried telegraphed only savoir faire; he was noted for the trail of brokenhearted supermodels in his wake. Perhaps it was just the tan (susceptible as I am to them), but he possessed an electric sort of energy, a life force; if you were to knock him down, it seems, he'd pop right back up again. The Playboy's office had nothing in it but an empty black table and two black sofas; he always appeared to be simply stopping by, coming or going somewhere, in transit. And he was, most of the time, since almost every photograph in the magazine was shot by him.

Also sometimes in the very same office was Grand-père, a white-haired, somewhat enfeebled Frenchman who'd launched *Elle* in the United States with the Playboy. Though he did not seem to have responsibility for much, his position was technically higher than the Playboy's; he had an imperious air and was inclined toward starched gingham shirts with carefully knotted ties. When they were both around, the two of them chuckled together all day in the big office, calling each other affectionate names ("my little hen") and thinking up political schemes. Grand-père also spent a lot of time sleeping; at one point, he had a special assistant who would slip a red pillow under his neck at the appointed time.

At the other end of the building, the stunning corner office belonged to Above the Fray, the American editor in chief who, too, was charming and short and fiftyish, sexy in the way you might expect Carly Simon's sister would be. Her intelligence was palpable, her curiosity about other people truly magnetic. She dressed in beautiful suits and beautiful shoes that reflected all she'd learned in her many years in magazines rather than a particular enchantment with fashion. Her black table was covered with articles being edited, always a gorgeous bunch of flowers, and an enormous vial (about the size of a picnic thermos) of Bulgari Eau au Thé, which, if you were familiar enough, you could spritz on from time to time. Her sofas each had embroidered pillows sent by Manolo Blahnik; our meetings were always held on the sofas, facing each other.

Above the Fray's office was surrounded by features people on either side; my office sat directly between features and art—equidistant from the two corner offices.

The two sides loathed each other. Magazines are usually dictatorships, with the editor in chief as the despot (friendly or not), but at *Elle* most of the power, at the end of the day, was consolidated in the hands of the Playboy, mostly because his pictures appeared not only in American *Elle*, but in the forty-odd editions of *Elle* that appear in countries around the world, an enormously efficient state of affairs for Hachette in terms of finances. Fashion shoots are very expensive things; the *Vogue* in Japan does all its own shoots, as does the one in Brazil.

Marketing

Positioned as it was like a giant emphatic exclamation point at the corner of her desk, Above the Fray's bottle of Bulgari perfume made everyone in the office want Bulgari perfume very badly. Co-worker after co-worker would casually drop by my office with some stunningly elaborate reason why, if there was any way I could, perhaps, just rustle up a bottle of . . . Bulgari . . . because they . . . Just as fashion designers send closets full of clothes to movie stars, perfume companies should send big bottles of perfume to CEOs across the nation. A nice big perfume makes an awfully good paperweight, one that could well be worth its weight in platinum in terms of sales to underlings.

Hachette smartly saved zillions by reprinting the Playboy's photographs in all the different editions.

While Hachette's management was American, the ownership, in Paris, was French. Why exactly the Playboy and Grand-père always hated the editor in chief (they had deposed a string of American editors in chief before Above the Fray arrived), I don't know, exactly. I got an inkling once when I visited the South of France. All the ancient little villages in Provence are built atop hills, mountains, or outcroppings. Their towers, as a result, really tower. You look down on the flatlands all around and imagine someone, anyone, approaching and how you might spear or cannonball or hot-oil them as they attempted to reach you. It was all about protecting a fiefdom, always with an eye toward expansion.

All the gifts and front-row designations and free clothes in the fashion business further aggravated the already intense

Editorial Integrity

Another cost saver for Hachette: When the Playboy's pictures arrived in the office, no art director—or even the editor in chief—ever, ever said they were all wrong. Too contrast-y, overexposed, slightly blurry? We all nodded our heads in agreement that the pictures were fantastically gorgeous, and into the magazine they went. That's power for you. And to be honest, if I were running a publishing company, I'd lean more in that direction than most of them do. Every day, at magazines besides *Elle*, they throw zillions of dollars out the window just so everything will be exactly, precisely right. But it's subjective—no one knows what *is* exactly, precisely right.

If I were Condé Nast or Hearst, I'd hire an editor to produce a random magazine cobbled together with all the rejected shoots and stories from all the magazines I owned. I bet it would be pretty good.

power struggle. Woe to the editor who received something flashy—say, the Prada skis that arrived in the fashion people's offices one Christmas—that the Playboy did not. If a designer kissed Above the Fray first at a party or a fashion show, there was sure to be some sort of retaliation the next day. If Fashionista, the fearsome fashion director, had too many flowers on her desk one day, she'd find herself iced out of an important meeting later that afternoon. Tribute was key.

It was not just about power, though. The French and the Americans had very different ideas of what the magazine should be. The fashion pictures in *Elle* are French and sexy. The models are pouting, leaping, pigeon-toe-posed objects, and there's just no way around it. The Frenchmen were forever

It Wasn't Me! I Swear!

The makeup you see on the covers of most magazines, or on fashion pages, is rarely the work of the beauty editor. Beauty editors produce articles about beauty; while they're responsible for the look of the pictures in the beauty articles, the fashion team—makeup artists, stylists, fashion editors, art directors, and photographers—produce the rest.

gunning for entire issues devoted to butts, and for more plastic surgery articles. They dressed the models in practically nothing, messed up their hair, and smudged eyeliner everywhere.

The articles, on the other hand, were much smarter and more interesting than your average women's magazine: brilliant art and book criticism, top-notch reporting on everything from economics to open-heart surgery to traveling in Bhutan, insightful meditations on health issues, love, intimacy. Even in the beauty section, there was no getting away with the usual "It's winter! Put on some moisturizer!" articles you find in most magazines. There always had to be an idea Above the Fray had never heard of, and your case had to be bolstered by experts from the NIH *and* Isaac Mizrahi *and* Nan Kempner. We interviewed philosophers about beauty, asked the country's top lawyers what makeup they wore (not much, P.S.), and convinced a brilliant gay rights activist to write about having her hair dyed.

You could get whiplash very quickly bouncing back and forth between the American, "thinking woman's" *Elle*—the articles—and the French, sexpot *Elle*—the pictures. I always wondered what the readers who loved the insightful journalism made of the makeup-spattered harlots prancing on the beach and what the readers who loved the prancing harlots made of the picture-free tracts on intimacy.

It was not that the editorial side was uninterested in sex; this was far from the case. There were endless discussions of male beauty on the American, editorial side. We were forever publishing "sexiest man" lists and thinking up articles on the topic. The features types would gather round, and I would be brought in for my beauty expertise, and we would discuss: They were all for the "thinking woman's" man. Liam Neeson headed every list, much to my dismay.

We had JFK Jr. working on his new magazine, *George,* in our conference room, and he never even came up. It was always a Liam Neeson or Ralph Fiennes. I'd bring up Keanu and they'd laugh uproariously. I finally put my foot down when Ted Koppel and Henry Kissinger made the list. "Ted Koppel and Henry Kissinger are valid human beings, but they are ugly human beings!" I burst out. "We aren't putting Margaret Thatcher on our cover!"

"But Margaret Thatcher is a horrible human being," the editors admonished. They could not be made to understand.

Heterosexual men who were not French, not JFK Jr., or not carrying out high-level political shenanigans were in short supply—heterosexual men in general are a rare thing at women's fashion magazines—so the ones who did exist got a lot of play. We all loved Dave, the muscle-bound art associate from Buffalo, the sort of guy who appears normally as a mythical figure in an old Bruce Springsteen song but was somehow plunked down, improbably, in fashion central.

Dave was that ever-rarer sort of man who's unafraid to tell you you look great. For the most part, either men are worried that you'll think they're in love with you and they'll look stupid or they go the other direction into that aggressive, "hey, baby, you know you want it" vibe that gives their entire gender a bad name. So we all paraded past Dave at least seventy times a day, glowering as he gazed appreciatively at others, blooming like riotous azaleas when he remarked on that skirt or those boots that you'd put on that morning, hoping against hope that Dave might notice them.

I and several others went so far as to join the company softball team (of which Dave was naturally a member). I cannot speak for the others, but the ridiculousness of my joining any sort of softball team, let alone a corporate-sponsored softball team, is just beyond. Under normal circumstances, I'd rather chew glass, or perhaps calculate pi, than play softball. Not only did I go, and actually attempt to pitch, hit, etc. (with little success, unsurprisingly), I even attended the after-game beerfests, invariably held at foul, luck-o'-the-Irish-themed bars that under normal circumstances I'd sooner chew glass, calculate pi, *and* play softball than set foot in. All to no avail. Dave, to our collective chagrin, was a gentleman.

Fortunately, for my first year, as the senior beauty editor, the dramas I endured were of that variety; I remained blissfully unaware of the high-level French/American contretemps. I had a boss, the beauty director (long ago, if you were the editor of something, they called you the editor, but now, in a grade-inflation-y way, *director* is the fancier term; to me, director sounds like some middle-management cog forever trapped by the three sage-colored half walls of his particleboard cubicle), who navigated the politics—so I simply did my job.

Truth in Stereotyping

At one point, my friend Adam (then Dave's boss) embarked on a Pygmalion project to transform Dave, to make him understand fashion. "He'll make so much more money in his career if he can just figure this out," Adam theorized. Out came stacks of Italian *Vogue* and *Nylon* and *The Face*. He pointed out things like sleeve lengths and bias cuts and heel shapes. He drilled, he quizzed, he reviewed. And Dave tried, he really did. But after several weeks of hard work, he remained immune to the subtleties of Versace versus Marc Jacobs; the cut of a Balenciaga moved him not at all; Kate Moss and Christy Turlington remained generic—if hot—chicks whose names he could never quite seem to place.

In a related, almost converse incident, Adam once made a new friend at Starbucks. They agreed to go out; she seemed vivacious and funny and smart. He was thrilled (he'd just moved to a new town and had no friends). When they met up, he used the word *peplum* to describe what was great about her dress. Her face fell.

"You're gay?" she cried, guessing correctly. *"Peplum?!"*

The office itself was not especially glamorous, except, as Gary and his visiting seventeen-year-old brother discovered, on "new model day," when hundreds of hopefuls would crowd the reception area. Otherwise we might have been a slightly down-at-the-heels management consultancy or some sort of governmental agency: white walls, gray cubicles, peeling paint here and there, horrifyingly lit bathrooms.

I was deep into the words side; I wrote articles and more articles. Above the Fray was brilliant; I learned more from her about writing and working for magazines than anyone else, ever. A few articles with her editing marks all over them are worth more than a graduate degree in journalism. She also took me under her wing in ways it took me years to fully realize: Not even a month into my job at *Elle*, she assigned me a story that involved getting to know Evelyn Lauder, perhaps the most influential woman in the entire beauty industry.

Above the Fray gave me my own column, called "Godfrey's Guide," which not only helped me develop my voice, but also had my name splashed across it every month. "You've been smart," Bobbi Brown once said to me. "You put your name all over everything. Then you're irreplaceable. My friend Ellen Tracy and I were just talking about that over lunch." I owe an enormous debt to Above the Fray.

I sat in a cubicle surrounded by the features people. Features are articles not pertaining to fashion or beauty, and they have

*Red Lipstick: The Unvarnished Truth

You know how it's always claimed that everyone can wear red, you just have to find the one that's right for your skin tone? Lie. A makeup company sent me the coolest long flat metal box, packed, ammunition style, with forty bulletlike lipsticks in every conceivable shade of red. Every morning, I would try on a new one and parade around the office, hoping that this, at last, would be it. A panel of experts including now world-famous *Lucky* editor Kim France (then the features editor at *Elle*) would weigh in; regretfully, the results were always the same: "Sorry, honey." Just think how much money I would've had to waste on this experiment had I chosen another career.

their own harder-news, more journalistic sort of glamour, though aside from the occasional celebrity encounter, their lives are generally less glamorous than those of the fashion people. The research and copy people (who toil over the articles of others, generally wishing they, too, got to write the articles) were adjacent. We all laughed and joked and ordered in lunch and tried on lipstick,* oblivious to the draconian machinations going on just over our heads.

Not entirely oblivious: We heard the screams coming from the fashion department down the hall.

I (like everyone else) avoided the fashion department like the plague. Fashion was ruled by the aforementioned Fashionista, who governed with an iron fist. In retrospect, her more frightening qualities may have been amplified by the fact that she was being tortured by both the French and the Americans; both had very strong opinions about fashion.

No matter what department, though, everyone was busy angling, all the time, kissing up to this or that person, trying to cut that one off at the knees. I just smiled and did my section of the magazine and handed out beauty products as liberally as I could. At one point, the words people had more power than usual; I got the job of beauty director, and my more French-associated boss got the boot.

Of course, it didn't happen just like that. When you work for an editor—any editor—a big part of your job is producing ideas for stories. No good ideas, eventually, adds up to no job. So I produced ideas, furiously. I sent them to both my boss and her boss. Like Fashionista, my boss was under constant stress between the French and the Americans and was perhaps already worried about her job for reasons that were far above my level of understanding, but eventually she wrote me a memo instructing me to stop producing ideas.

Then, naturally, I had an idea that simply could not go unmentioned: A new, enormous supergym was coming to New York from Los Angeles, and no one knew about it yet except me and the person who'd tipped me off. We would scoop even *Vogue*, which we rarely did (such was our rivalry that the beauty editor of *Vogue* and I had a cabal of sorts, wherein we used to call each other every month, just to make sure we weren't running any of the same products in our new beauty items page, so as to avoid the rage of higher-ups on both sides).

I was incredibly excited, and I wrote a memo all about it, thinking that the idea was so important that the "no more ideas" rule would be overlooked, just this once.

It was not. My boss screamed at me in front of everyone; every head in the sea of cubicles that was features, copy, research, and beauty turned in horror. Injustice, perceived or actual, really sends me over the edge. I cried all day: I had many appointments, so I cried in the cab from one appointment to the next, collecting myself as I paid the fare and explaining to everyone that I had horrible allergies.

The next day the managing editor, Above the Fray's number two, whispered, "Come with me," and spirited me through a labyrinthine series of hallways to an office I had never been in before. Behind the desk was a small, sprightly woman with dark hair. "Tell her what happened yesterday," instructed the managing editor. I assumed I was being fired. I was terrified, but I told.

The next day, moving men came for my boss's things and took them to a new floor while she was out at lunch; we were later told that she now worked for Hachette's custom publishing division.

(Epilogue: *Vogue*, of course, ended up with the super-gym

story—they did a huge, fantastic feature shot by Helmut Newton, with Nadia Auermann contorting herself in all sorts of glamorous positions amid the gleaming machinery, atop the spectacular roof deck.)

Now, of course, they needed to replace my boss. "Who do you know in the beauty industry, Jean, who would be a really, really good beauty editor?" Above the Fray implored. "You've got to know someone." She interviewed and interviewed, and no one worked. She would ask at least once a day. "There's got to be someone!"

It drove me insane. I could not believe she could be so insensitive or so blind. Here she loved my work, I knew the beauty industry . . . At last, a wise compatriot looked at me as we emerged from yet another meeting where Above the Fray was again bemoaning our lack of a beauty director: "Jean, you've got to at least say you're *interested.*"

After our next meeting about purple eye shadow or whatever it may have been, she again brought up the issue, and somehow, somehow I managed to squeak out a "Well, what about me?" as I snuck out the door.

"Well," she said, regarding me with a quizzical eye (she knew the pressures that one step up the ladder would expose me to, while I, of course, did not), "I didn't think you would want it." All those dumb things they say in salesmanship manuals and sex advice books about asking for what you want? True.

Of course, that wasn't all there was to it; I had to interview with the publisher and be run by the Frenchmen, but amazingly, no one objected to the somewhat questionable terms of my ascent or to my marked lack of experience on staff at a fashion magazine (I'd been there a year). I got it.

I got off to a rough start as the beauty director: One of the first stories I did was an interview with Elizabeth Hurley. It went with some pictures of her on the beach in East Hampton—writhing on the dunes in a tight, peacock-colored Gucci pantsuit—taken, naturally, by the Playboy. The story came out to great fanfare; I was encouraged.

Leaving one night, I got to the elevator just as the Playboy and Grand-père reached it. We went in. "!@#$%^GlElizabeth-HurleyFFHJ^%$#@!" said the Playboy. He was speaking English, but not well.

I looked at him. "Yes!" I said brightly.

They both looked confused and affronted. Grand-père tried to explain: "!@#$%^GelHElizabethHurleyFHHJ^*&*!"

"Yes!" I exclaimed again, beaming hopefully. Just as the elevator reached the ground floor, the French-inflected words began to sort themselves out in my mind, and I realized what the Playboy had actually said: "Your name was bigger than mine on the Elizabeth Hurley story!" To which I'd cheerfully replied, twice, "Yes!"

Shortly after, I was dispatched to Paris—along with all the scary fashion operatives—for the shows. I arrived in Paris, and all the *Elle* fashion editors, still loyal to my predecessor, wouldn't speak to me beyond a stony "Sorry, there's no room in this car."

Paris is an impenetrable maze unless you're familiar with it, so to get around to fashion shows, you need a car service. Especially because one show will be at one location at 2:00 p.m., and the next show will be completely across the city and supposedly start at 3:00 p.m. The 2:00 p.m. show, of course, never starts on time—you're lucky if it finally gets going at 3:30, so you're out at 4:00, the sun is setting, and you were supposed to be across town an hour ago.

Interview Beauty Tips

I know, it's all about the work, not your looks. But I—a very dark horse for various jobs throughout my career—have my tips anyway.

1. **The person who's interviewing you is the most attractive person in the world.** This is less grotesque than it sounds. If you're the type who's got all sorts of running commentary going through your head *(that was a stupid thing to say, why'd I say that, I wonder how much money I could ask for, when is this going to be over, I wonder how I look . . .)*, focus your attention instead on whatever you think is the most attractive feature of the person across the table and really think hard about how lovely he or she is. Somehow, whether that person can actually read minds or your general attitude toward that person becomes more relaxed or more focused—who knows? But try it.

2. **No green eye shadow, etc.** If ever there was a moment for the natural look, both makeup and hairwise, it would be the big interview. Nothing says "grifter" like dark, sticky lip gloss and a pair of false eyelashes. Anyway.

3. **If within the realm of possibility, wear something new and fabulous.** For my interview with the publisher (money guy) of *Elle*, I purchased a gorgeous red silk striped jacket—it made me think of Morocco or, more succinctly, a sophisticated Frenchwoman who'd picked up her jacket when she was in Morocco because she was so fantastically chic—I've never worn it since. But I felt great in it at the time, and that's all that counts.

   The other nice thing about something new is you don't have to iron it. When I iron something, it ends up looking far worse than when I started.

Elevator Authority Anxiety

There's something about an authority figure in an elevator that sends me completely over the edge. In fact, I think top publishing operatives like Anna Wintour, James Truman, Si Newhouse, and the like should get together and write a big coffee table book detailing the many ridiculous things that have been said to them—or performed before them—as they've attempted to ride up the elevator in silence. I'm a fairly restrained person, and the elevator gets to me; I'd be interested to read what the less disciplined might do if given a chance.

And though you'd think the French would be cooler, as a population, with regard to fashion shows, this is not the case. They are all desperate to go, and they line up outside the shows, dressed to kill, and they hiss and elbow their way toward you, determined to wrest a ticket from your Ugly American hands.

I made my way through the melee and at last sat down at Valentino, my first show ever. I was in the third row; I crossed my legs like the other editors, took a swig of the free Evian from the gift bag, and settled in. Grand-père waved me over.

He had sent a folder of magazine clippings to me when I first got the beauty director position. "Grand-père likes these layouts," the assistant had mentioned cryptically.

Now, at Valentino, Grand-père beckoned me over to introduce me to the editor in chief of French *Elle*. "Zees ees the woman who makes zee layouts that I show you," he said pointedly, his smile turning to a scowl. "Now zat you meet her, maybe you stop throwing zem in zee trash can!" They both turned their backs on me.

Everyone heard the nasty, humiliating exchange, and the incident seemed to solidify their general impression that I would not be lasting long. The debonair publisher (head salesperson, money person) of the magazine thankfully did not hear it. He arrived late, slid into his front-row seat, spotted me in the third row—and, because (being American) he had a frosty relationship with the French, waved me forward. "Sit next to me," he said. "They can't put *Elle* in the third row!" He elbowed me halfway through: "What's with Linda's breasts? You're the beauty editor—is that plastic surgery?" If you've got someone to stage-whisper through a fashion show with, you're okay.

As it turned out, the publisher had beauty advertisers on his schedule for lunch, so he told me to meet him later at La Stresa, the legendary Italian restaurant in the 18th arrondissement. I had a show and a lunch in St. Germain de Pres before that, but I of course agreed. No editor had space in her car, naturally, so I had to get there on my own; I made it through the show (everything was late, *naturellement*) and somehow managed to scramble to the first lunch. I had an hour. The French perfume executive ordered glass after glass of wine and course after course of foie gras and steak *frites* and *salade* (as my heart pounded louder and I ground my teeth more furiously) as the clock ticked ever closer to 2:00 p.m., when I was supposed to be across town at Stresa. At 1:50, I finally blurted that I had a show and couldn't be late. I dashed out the door and broke into a headlong run—I ran from the Left Bank to the Right, past the Champs-Elysées and all the way to the 18th in fifteen minutes. La Stresa, La Stresa, the appropriately named La Stresa. I thought I was going to have a heart attack right there.

The maître d' nodded when I said the name of my publisher and quickly led me to one of the restaurant's several inner sanctums. On the way in, we passed the Playboy and Grand-père in deep conversation with . . . Catherine Deneuve, looking as Catherine Deneuve–y as possible: upswept hair, kohl-rimmed eyes, the palest pink suit. They obviously hadn't seen that the *Elle* publisher was in the next room, so I appeared to be glamorous enough to get in there all on my own. They hailed me over to their table. "Catrine, zees ees our *directrice de beauté*," said Grand-père, beaming at me as if he were indeed my proud grandfather. My apparent glamour canceled out all the morning's trouble. "Her name is Jeanne Godfrey-June— she ees brilliant!"

"*Enchanté*," said Catherine, smiling and sipping her Châteauneuf-du-Pape.

And like that, I was in.

Perception is everything, especially when you're perceiving fabulousness. For instance, I assumed, on that trip, that the hotel we all stayed in was one of those clean but unremarkable, convenient places that companies put their employees in; the Frenchmen themselves were in another hotel, which I assumed was the Paris-luxe one. I am always impressed by the luxury of hotels, because I spent my childhood yearning to stay in one as the rain dripped onto my sleeping bag and the wind blew heartlessly through the tarp in the subzero weather. A Motel 6, with its cellophane-wrapped plastic drink cups and its thin rectangles of harsh white soap, is still a site of impossible glamour for me, to this day. While this wasn't a Motel 6, my excitement over being in it was my usual excitement: In a hotel! Not camping!

Although my room was large, I had never stayed in Paris,

When You're Up, You're Up, and When It's Over, So Are You

Perhaps *Elle* was an extreme example of the fragility and vicissitudes of success and failure, but I think this point is key to happiness in any job: Yes, when you're hot everybody loves you, and when you're not, a big bunch of them are going to forget you in the blink of an eye. It's not about you, it's about human nature. Bitterness is the ugliest fate imaginable, so give it up.

except in a youth hostel, so I assumed this was Parisian par for the course. While my large marble bathroom had Hermès toiletries in it, I again thought, Well, those French.

Several years later, when Hachette made several modest cost-cutting measures and we got a new hotel, I realized that I'd wasted all my precious moments at the Hotel Le Bristol (one of the priciest places to stay on earth, the spot where Audrey Hepburn and Cary Grant stalk one another in *Charade*) thinking it was just average.

Of course, the battle wasn't entirely won yet. Not even my thrilling triumph at La Stresa moved the fashion editors. No, that took an actual beauty moment:

The height of chic in Paris then (and now) was neither a lipstick shade nor a new perfume. It was reaching into your Hermès bag from your front-row seat, extracting an impossibly tiny cell phone, calling the Chinese restaurant Davé, and having your close personal friend Davé say yes when you asked for a reservation.

Models

Even though models are genetic freaks and paid millions solely for their camera friendliness, and even though they're then piled with makeup and specially lit to make them thousands of times *more* beautiful, it's still not enough, and magazines spend many hours and dollars digitally enhancing the supposedly already perfect model. The all-time low was a *Bazaar* cover where they felt compelled to shave off so much of Cindy Crawford's absolutely perfect (I've seen them, and they are) arms and thighs that she looked like a paper doll that had been soaked in water and was starting simply to dissolve.

So again: Nothing, nothing in the world is going to make you look like that magazine cover, because people don't actually look like that.

While I had managed to wangle a seat (if not front row) at the shows, the bag and the close personal friendship with Davé (pronounced, Dav-AY, lest you confuse him with Dave, the lone heterosexual in the *Elle* art department) remained tantalizingly out of reach. So when a group of friends-of-Davé invited me to dinner, I leapt at the chance. Once there, I marveled at the crowd—models in filmy thrift shop negligees and moldy car coats, Italians in cashmere, editors in black—and wondered how to strike up a conversation with the all-important Davé, who flitted around the room from Beautiful to Powerful and back again.

In the restroom, I noted a lavish outpouring of rose-infused potpourri—something I'd previously associated with mauve-obsessed Home Depot regulars but now instantly saw was

Murphy's Law (Model's Version)

Sad to say, models can't be categorized as either dumb or smart. There's about the same variation as in the general population, though I will say this: Too much choice (since you're a model, you can have anyone, correct?) is clearly a bad thing when it comes to men. Your typical superhot, $10,000-a-day model ends up with a not-so-hot, often ill-tempered man destined to cheat on her or descend into substance abuse.

headed for a major, Gucci-esque resurgence. I'd found, at last, the beauty angle.

"Tell me, Davé," I said, finding him deep in the swirl of steamed dumplings and onetime celebrities. "Potpourri?" A banal opening, it might seem. But a beauty discussion greases social wheels like nothing else. People who won't let on with their first names collapse into chatterboxes, detailing their bad hair, their expensive moisturizer, their travails against acne.

Davé, too, had lots to say. "I dry my own roses!" he gushed, taking me under his arm. "I scent zem with rose extract, you know, zis special blend from L'Artisan Parfumer. . . ."

Seeing me chatting so casually with my new friend Davé, two of the formerly frosty *Elle* editors sidled up to me immediately. "Jean! We didn't see you! We're sitting right over there!"

Fashion people are the snottiest people on earth, bar none, and even they can't resist a beauty angle.

Hair and Makeup "Trends"

You can tell which designers are closet misogynists by the "statements" they make with hair and makeup on their runways. Lovely cut-on-the-bias evening dresses notwithstanding, patent-leather stick-on eyebrows are just a big dead giveaway. Eyebrows are a particularly egregious thing to screw with, I think; there was a year when they shaved off the models' brows completely, making them all look like potential suicides. Great cones sculpted out of hair, pointing from the models' heads like so many 1950s-starlet breasts, is another common offense, particularly in Paris. Or the work of Mondrian, interpreted literally onto the face with big squares of bright makeup painted right over the gorgeous models' billions-of-dollars-a-day features. There's rarely any information to be gleaned from these looks, aside from the fact that they're probably there to distract the viewer from otherwise boring or tortured clothes.

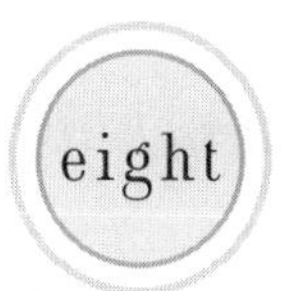

Directrice de Beauté

Back in the office, I soon realized that the single rung on the ladder I'd managed to ascend made everything very, very different: I no longer sat in a cubicle. I had an office with an assistant sitting outside of it, waiting to help me. My phone rang off the hook with PR and marketing people, previously uninterested in me, now all desperate to take me to lunch. I had a clothing allowance, which is the single greatest perk ever invented. I've never been able to finagle one again, but while it lasted, I shopped in the relaxed, highest-quality-only, I'll-take-four-of-those-yes-in-all-the-colors way that I suppose only very rich women do. If I bought something that didn't work out, I said to myself, I get paid to make fashion mistakes, *paid.*

In addition, a whole new world of stress and politics revealed itself. I had meetings at both ends of the office and often found myself relaying messages between the French side and the American, never a pleasant task. While I remained calm by accepting the fact that I would eventually be fired in as brutal a way as possible, I navigated significant challenges: The Playboy did not have time to produce images for the beauty section, since he was busy with almost all of the fashion and all the covers besides. In addition, the makeup favored by the Playboy and his team, as I've mentioned, was mostly of the "I put on too much eyeliner and then he had his way with me" variety. Occasionally I could cull a beauty image from a fashion shoot he'd done—this would result in the instant approval of whatever I put on such pages—but most of the time, I had to have another photographer shoot the beauty pictures.

If they were too good, they'd never make it into the magazine. The Playboy would pronounce the shots awful and the photographer talentless, and he would, if I were lucky, produce some eyeliner-heavy, hopefully-in-focus outtakes from one of his fashion shoots. The trick was to produce pictures that were just pretty enough—but not so good they'd be cut.

There was also the Fashionista to consider: She still inspired more terror around the office than anyone else. When I arrived back from the collections, she summoned me to her office. I had done something she didn't like. Perhaps sitting in the front row at Valentino. "Jean Godfrey-June," she said in a high-pitched voice, "we really like you here, and we want you to succeed." She paused dramatically. "*We'd hate to see you fired.*" I'd been warned.

A few weeks later, I came back from a PR lunch to find my door closed and my assistant cowering behind it.

"Kate," I stammered.

"Close the door!" she demanded in a hoarse whisper. She'd been in the beauty closet, minding her own business, when suddenly in swept Fashionista, whom she'd never met. "Hair spray!" screamed Fashionista in a frenzy. "I need hair spray! I have a TV crew in my office!" Before Kate could even move, Fashionista snatched a bottle from the shelf and started spraying her hair furiously—with big puffy white clouds of mousse.

Because mousse is, as frequently promised, "as light as air," Fashionista had no idea that her head now swirled with snowy blobs, and she rushed out of the room before Kate could stop her, leaving a trail of white soft-serve-ish bits on the carpet behind her.

"I'm going to be fired," Kate wailed. "I don't think even you can help me." I told her to calm down, because I knew the truth: Kate was an assistant, an underling—so someone like Fashionista had no use for her and thus could not see her at all. Her lowness on the totem pole protected her like Harry Potter's Cloak of Invisibility. Kate ran right into Fashionista the next day, and Fashionista whooshed right past her, oblivious, *her* assistant scurrying behind her, scrambling to pick up the boxes and bags and fur coats left in her wake.

Fashionista herself had it rough, however. I was crammed in the elevator with a number of people one day, among them the Playboy and his model/editor/socialite wife (I'll call her Model Wife), who involved herself with the magazine wherever she could. Model Wife is one of those tanned, athletic, white teeth, blond hair American beauties, gorgeous in that friendly "hot girl next door" way. Model Wife looked over at him adoringly. "Playboy," she said, "maybe we should be nice to Fashionista again," flashing a toothy smile.

"Just for fun," he replied, smiling back.

It was that arbitrary. Even being in favor had its troubles. The Playboy and Model Wife loved Jack Russell terriers. So they purchased one for Fashionista for her birthday, which, of course, she had to accept cheerfully and then take care of, forever. Several key stylists also had Jack Russells, though whether they purchased them on their own or received them as gifts I'll never know.

Working with Above the Fray was incredible, as I've explained, but it was not easy: Turn in a lame article to her, and you were going to hear about it. Present not entirely thought out ideas at the editorial meeting and woe to you.

Beyond fashion, the French, and the Americans, there was an éminence grise to be placated: the dark-haired woman whom I'd told my sad tale of injustice to, who'd clearly been the reason my boss lost her job, whom here, despite her not-French background, I will refer to as Eminence Grise. Ostensibly Eminence Grise was a money person, an accountant sort, perhaps, who lived in a suburb in New Jersey and helped the magazine figure out its various financial and personnel issues. In reality, she secretly ruled the whole magazine, Americans *and* French (she almost always sided with the French) and eventually ruled not just us but several other Hachette titles as well.

Our last names were similar in such a way that we looked like the same person on the interoffice phone; I think that accident of fate was a powerful factor in my advancement at *Elle.* If someone looked down as they answered the phone and saw whom they thought it was (Eminence Grise), they practically jumped out of their skin. We'd laugh about it, of course, but the damage would have been done in terms of the way they perceived me.

Despite her Machiavellian treatment of many others—she seemed to relish firing people, for example, and once eagerly offered to fire a woman for me, a woman she herself had never even met—she was always nice to me and would help smooth things over if, for instance, the Playboy hated the photography or fashion was terrorizing me. Or if the demands of one of the many beauty-product-and-service-crazed wives—practically every man at Hachette had a spoiled, wealthy wife desperate for free products, haircuts, and spa trips—were getting out of hand.

Eminence Grise was always teaming up with the French against Above the Fray. One day, they decided to fire the art director. (Above the Fray had hired her.) Instead of just firing the poor art director, they hired a new one (Adam, who was ostensibly there to work on something else, and who, it should be noted, eventually became one of my closest friends) and had him begin working on layouts at a desk in front of her office. When the art director just kept working, Eminence Grise was eventually dispatched; she slammed the old art director's door shut, and we could literally hear screams coming from inside. God knows what actually occurred, but when the door opened, the old art director was packing her bags, quickly.

This sort of torture is not endemic to *Elle* magazine, I should note: It's what fashion magazines everywhere are all about—You wore a gross outfit? Mixed up the sushi order? Mispronounced Gaultier? Sorry.

Adam's arrival sent waves of fresh hope through the desperate-for-men *Elle* operatives. Adam is wildly smart, funny, and charming, not to mention shockingly handsome; straight he is most definitely not, but both his manner and his penchant for superbutch biker outfits leave this question open to viewers' interpretation.

We became friends despite the fact that at our first meeting I popped an M&M into his mouth (perhaps he was yawning), and he recoiled, stricken. I might as well have fed him a tablet of anthrax or plutonium; he was and remains terrified of fat. Like an overgrown teenager, he is thus compelled to consume enormous amounts of (as fat-free as possible) food in order to get enough calories. He often ordered two or three lunches just to get by, a trait I found endearing.

That and the way he reacted when I inadvertently crossed him, complaining about something or other to the all-powerful

Eminence Grise. Like Fashionista, he summoned me to his office, but he was much more charming and did not threaten to fire me.

"You don't have to tell on the art department when you need something, Jean Godfrey-June," he said, looking me in the eye with his far-more-beautiful eyes. "We love you, Jean Godfrey-June, there's no reason not to just come in here and sort it out."

My office was filled with fashion girls, research assistants, and features people, all passing innocently through—just like the Bulgari—just stopping by and somehow winding their way around to, "So, do you think he's straight?"

Adam, being in art, had to contend with the French/American standoff much more directly than I. Being male, he also heard what they really felt. "We have it so easy, working for a women's magazine," one of the French observed one day. "Women, they don't understand—you can give them anything and they'll read it. Think if we had to work for *Time*, or *Newsweek*, how hard we would have to work." Another time, one of them had made a change on something Above the Fray had done, and Adam pointed it out to them: "She's never going to go for this."

"Oh no, she is a woman! She won't get it—women are too stupid for this kind of thing."

We cemented our friendship at a cringe-inducing *Elle* party in the Hamptons. It was called "Get Your Jeans Off!" and involved demicelebs each decorating his or her own pair of jeans, which were then to be auctioned off for charity at the party, held in fancy white tents on the polo fields. The Playboy wrangled plenty of supermodels to Bedazzle up their jeans; Fashionista wrangled movie stars, who in turn, together with the Playboy, wrangled art world operatives.

A select group of *Elle* staffers were "the crowd." We had to show, so that the party appeared buzzing and chic to the real invitees. Slip dresses were still the height of cool, and I had purchased a yellow one, but after several try-on-abort moments in front of the mirror, trying to make it work—I really cannot work a yellow, no matter what lip gloss shade I choose to counter, no matter how fabulous the accessories. Standing in a crumpled pile of clothing, I finally resigned myself to this fact once and for all. Instead, I pieced together an old, somewhat torn actual black slip—one I'd bought, specifically to wear under another skirt, for $5 in New Orleans—with a white T-shirt. The trend, with a twist! I was triumphant.

As I was running out the door to meet Adam (we were driving out together), my baby-sitter clutched my arm: "Mrs. June, Mrs. June, you . . . you forgot to put on your skirt." I tried to explain that no, that really *was* my skirt; the baby-sitter was unconvinced. Out of context, fashion really does make no sense.

Adam, too, contended with fashion challenges, so we arrived late, but not late enough; it was small talk small talk small talk, with land mines of trouble lying ready to explode in your face at every turn. People were on edge.

"OmigodyourskirtIsthatMiuMiu?" queried Fashionista as my kitten heels sank into the muddy grass.

"Uh . . . ?" I replied hopefully.

In swooped Adam. "Vintage," he said. "Isn't it fabulous?"

Everyone was anxious. There were the Playboy and Model Wife, looking tanned and strained. Eminence Grise and her husband, two suburban New Jersey fish out of water. A movie-star couple, looking vaguely affronted, deep in conversation with an uncomfortable Julian Schnabel. The models chatted

Vintage

The "vintage" excuse for items from the Salvation Army (as opposed to the trillion-dollar Ossie Clark/Valentino/Balenciaga offerings at true "vintage" stores like Lily et Cie, where the stars go to find an outfit no one else will be wearing) is the fashion equivalent of Maybelline Great Lash or perhaps a really great self-tanning job. All gain, no pain.

overenthusiastically into the *Access Hollywood* cameras. There's something so unfun about a party just for show like that.

The jeans weren't selling. It's hard enough trying to find a pair of jeans you like in real life, but each pair here was in a specific size, either tiny-supermodel or large-older-man-who-likes-supermodels. And then, of course, they were Bedazzled and paint splattered within an inch of their lives. And you were supposed to want to pay thousands of dollars for them. Even the oceans of cosmopolitans or sake-tinis or whatever the poor waiters were serving couldn't shake things up; panic began to creep into the proceedings, and the various artists began bidding for their own jeans, lest a low-selling price reflect something about their ascending or descending position in the world at large.

Adam and I resorted to my party trick of last resort, which I had perfected with my friend Susan in college at frat parties: pretending to talk. "Uh-huh!" says one person.

"Yeah, I know," says the other. "Really."

"That's the thing, right?"

"It *is* like that, you know."

The Cure for Boring Parties, Part Two

Beyond faking a conversation, which is funny but gets old, Susan and I discovered a way to have a good time at the dullest parties (it works only if you barely know anyone): Think of the funniest name you can—we leaned toward the trailer-trashier names like Tammy Jo, but Henrietta and Bertha are good, too—anything that will make you personally laugh, and write it on your name tag. Parties full of salespeople or fraternity brothers—any group that's been trained to repeat the name of the person they're speaking with over and over—make especially happy hunting grounds. "So where were you from, Tammy Jo?"

"So, Tammy Jo, what are you majoring in?"

The trick is to appear just animated enough; too much and you both dissolve in laughter, and the jig is up.

There is a famous American designer who, I found out over the course of several interviews, is a true master of this technique and doesn't even need a partner to make it work. While I was speaking to him, he sounded as if he were revealing incredibly personal, very smart, important, and earthshaking things. I scribbled notes furiously, went through tape after tape of it all, and when I played it back to write the article, I found nothing but "Uh-huh, yeah . . . well, the thing of it is . . . it's like *that*, you know, and it's all *about* that." It's very David Mamet (believe it or not, this actually happened to me twice), and my article ended up being about the amazing perfumes, clothes, etc., the designer had created and not, as I was hoping, about the true soul of the designer himself. The only questions with clear, reprintable answers were those on which he'd agreed to talk with me. It's genius and it's as it should be—a justified "none of your business" in the most pleasant, unconfrontational way possible. He could give lessons to all the poor celebrities who go on about their sex lives like flophouse trannies at the Laundromat.

"Come on, guys! Aren't you going to bid on something?" Model Wife interrupted sharply. Along with watching her flock of Jack Russells, getting her coffee, and calling in clothes/beauty products galore for her, the *Elle* staff did an enormous amount for the Playboy's wife; Adam was often called upon to squire her around to social events the Playboy was unwilling to attend, introduce her to people like Ross Bleckner, and pay for dinner after. I was often called upon to help her with her articles for *Top Model*, a brief publishing exercise Hachette went through for which she was the editrix.

"Bids?" she asked again, smiling.

"Of course, Model Wife, we just can't decide which jeans we want," Adam assured her in his cool, charming way.

"Adam really wants the Julian Schnabel ones," I added.

Eminence Grise and her husband cornered us to register their disgust at a sex scene in a novel by Above the Fray's prominent, wildly talented significant other. "I really, really, can't imagine the kind of person who would . . . *write* such a thing," droned the husband. He regarded my skirt suspiciously. "I mean, it kind of makes you want to throw up."

Eminence Grise nodded ponderously, then raised her face to us dramatically. "He wouldn't let me read it," she said. "Wouldn't. Let. Me. It's *that* awful."

There really was nowhere to turn. The party went on and

on and on, and our fake conversation looped like bad house music as we circulated from cluster to cluster of unsettled party-goers. As the sun began to set and "record prices" for the jeans were being shouted over the loudspeaker by Model Wife, we slipped away.

Adam was of course starving when we finally emerged from the horror. But the prospect of a fancy Hamptons boîte, bustling with the same types we'd just escaped, was too much to bear. We drove and drove and ended up in a bar strikingly reminiscent of the one in *The Accused.* We sat down, and as the somewhat menacing atmosphere began to sink in, I noticed several possible psychopaths/Harley-Davidson kingpins, their eyes trained hungrily on my slip, which, pre-torn as it was, must have seemed especially "she asked for it." Adam, seemingly oblivious, ordered four grilled-not-fried chicken breast entrées and devoured them, while I picked at a single chicken breast and ate french fries, glancing about nervously.

"Oh, don't worry," Adam mumbled through the chicken breast. "I can kill anyone. Really. I'll kill 'em."

You can't not love a person who resolutely believes that if push comes to shove, he's fully capable of killing his opponents and that to do so would be terrible but would not require a great amount of effort. And who orders his meals in triplicate.

○

At work, things escalated politically among Above the Fray, Eminence Grise, and the French Eminence Grise and the French upped the ante by deciding that from now on I and the fashion director would report not to Above the Fray, but to Eminence Grise herself (I of course still made every edit or art change Above the Fray asked for, as she knew much better

Big Money, Still Unmade

Eminence Grise once elucidated an important moneymaking opportunity for beauty companies, one that has yet to be capitalized on. "Jean," she said into the phone one day in her little-girl voice, "it's Eminence Grise. Can you come down to my office?" No scarier words were ever spoken, but down I went.

"I want to get my hair colored," she squeaked when I got there.

"Which salon—where do you want to go?" I asked.

"I already get my hair colored," she said, "but I don't have time anymore. Who has three hours every six weeks to waste in some salon? I want to know the perfect shade for me—from a box I can do at home." I sent her to experts at L'Oréal, who quickly gave her the perfect shade. If they could do that for your average woman, both rich and poor would flock to them, I suspect, and they'd make even more money than they already do.

than I, and I knew it). I thought this was the end, but again, strangely, it was not.

One thrilling development was that while Eminence Grise was my boss, she was also JFK Jr.'s boss. He would often be sitting in her office, finishing up, when I arrived, or he would arrive as I was finishing up, ready for his appointment. "Hi," I would say.

Because we shared the same terrifying/benevolent overlord, I always felt I knew JFK Jr. better than I actually did. At the same time, when I did see him *not* in the context of her office—say, in the elevator—some crazed voice inside me would insist that he was an impostor and not the real JFK Jr. Perhaps just some interloper who looked a lot like him. I would stare stonefacedly ahead as if I saw nothing; sometimes he'd say nothing, sometimes he'd say "hi."

He was referred to as "John" around the office, the way people in Hollywood say "Tom" or "Nicole." If he was not present when he was being referred to, higher-ups often called him "John-John." He was always carrying his bike or chaining it somewhere. Though handsome, JFK Jr. was not my type (I was clearly not his, either), so his presence in the conference room only glamorized me rather than implanting far-fetched hopes in my mind.

He would emerge from Eminence Grise's office as I went in, sighing heavily, beaten down in some way, and I'd think, Wow, that Eminence Grise is tough. If even JFK Jr. got this kind of treatment, someday my number'd be up, and it wasn't going to be pretty.

Instead, one day, the Playboy, as he seemed to do with all people in his life, turned on Eminence Grise, his ally in everything (by this point, Eminence Grise and the Playboy had done away with Above the Fray, Adam, several more art directors, *and* the impossible-to-unseat-but-they-managed Grand-père). Eminence Grise naturally couldn't believe the Playboy's betrayal; it seemed impossible. But like the countless, baffled, trusting supermodels and co-workers who found themselves entangled with the Playboy and then suddenly, brutally untangled, she, too, succumbed. *Elle* was harsh, there's no two ways about it.

Fashion Editor Lite

We all work at magazines in pursuit of some sort of glamour; as I've mentioned, the only truly glamorous fashion magazine workers are the fashion editors. That's just the way it is, and all beauty editors (myself included) delight in the occasional pretend fashion editor moment. *Elle* afforded me countless moments with top designers, which were, for the most part, similar to my many moments with celebrities and supermodels: You have your friendly bit of conversation, your handshake, and you move on. It doesn't add up to much—it's not like they're going to be calling you next week to dish about their ex-boyfriend or to borrow a cup of sugar.

There's a book called *I Dream of Madonna* that chronicles the many and varied dreams people have had about her (Rocco's mother, not Jesus'). I'm sure it'd be an easy thing to compile an *I Dream of George Clooney* or perhaps an *I Dream of Cheryl Tiegs* were they to discover a demand for such an item.

Me, I dream of Marc Jacobs. I started dreaming about him (he always appears as a very close friend) when I first moved to New York and he was the designer for Perry Ellis. We'd meet in coffee shops, laugh on street corners, hang out for long, lazy stretches at each other's apartments; I was

Me-Drag

Me-Drag: What someone might put on if they were dressing up as you—for Halloween, say, or some sort of roast. On genuinely glamorous types, you'd call it personal style.

My personal me-drag involves a choice of flippy skirt or corduroy pant, with either a sandal or a flip-flop, depending on the venue. Beautywise, the me-drag is even more restrictive: mascara (with a little liner—again, venue-dependent), self-tanner, and lip gloss that closely approximates my own lip color, except glossier and a bit more noticeable. While I like to think of myself as adventurous, this formula, in fact, never varies.

People talk about—really they deplore—falling into a style "rut," particularly when it leads mutton to dress as lamb. But if French *Vogue* editor Carine Roitfeld's outfit (with eyeliner) came stalking down the street by itself, you'd still know it was Carine (assuming you follow these things)—and you'd wish you were glamorous and decisive enough to dress so well (personal style is all about decision-making skills). If Andrée Putman's hair floated past, you'd say, "There goes Andrée Putman." If an ensemble put together by *Lucky* creative director Andrea Linett were suddenly to animate and come rushing by, you'd know whom to return it to. Technically, these women are in a rut. Just a very good rut—one that you'd never want to be "made over" out of by some beret-topped Hollywood stylist (berets are worn solely by Monica Lewinsky and Hollywood stylists, an odd but undeniable connection).

What I'm saying is, a little me-drag can be a very good thing.

there for him when no one understood grunge; he advised me to quit writing real estate copy and follow my dream: fashion magazines.

The only evidence I ever had that Marc Jacobs possessed

any reciprocal feelings of knowing *me* was at his first independent show, which he held glamorously at the Plaza hotel. Gilt-edged, red-velvet-upholstered chairs snaked the edge of the runway, and I was led, inexplicably, to a front-row seat directly across the way from Anna Wintour, the editor in chief of *Vogue* (I should note that beauty editors don't often rate the front or even the second row at fashion shows, as, of course, they have no power to put clothes into the magazine). In whisked more editors, heavy with importance yet chatting breezily with their seatmates, crossing their legs to reveal fabulous shoes, throwing down their million-dollar bags stuffed with thrilling papers and pencils and water bottles.

I sat in my seat, pretending to read my *Women's Wear Daily*, feeling like a sixteen-year-old who's managed to sneak into a bar and order a margarita undetected—scanning the room for someone who might suddenly appear, pointing a finger, I'd scream, "Wrong! Wrong! Get that one out of here!" The feel-

I do not know Karl Lagerfeld (not even in my dreams), but I admire him greatly nonetheless because I hear (as in hearsay) he throws out his underwear every day. You know?

And I think—too often—about the marketing possibilities surrounding the disposed-of tight whites? boxers? bikinis? I imagine sort of Versace-ish silk boxers, but I know that's all wrong—

Also hearsay are the tales of the vending machines in Japan that dispense the used underwear of prepubescent girls to otherwise dutiful salarymen; a vending machine with Karl's underwear in it, on the other hand, would draw crowds of eager prepubescent girls. (Chanel! Chanel!)

ing faded as the lights dimmed and the show started; the teenager in me began to sip, ever so tentatively, at the margarita. The models marched out, their hair shining and their makeup barely, prettily perceptible, the music romantic, the clothes gorgeous. What a world. And he—*my*—Marc Jacobs had invited me into it, with a front-row seat.

The next year, somewhat anticlimactically, I was back in the fifth row, but I didn't care. There's just something about a Marc Jacobs show.

But as the years (and the dreams) went on, reality continued to collide every so often with fantasy: I would encounter the actual Marc Jacobs, mostly backstage at fashion shows. I interviewed him on a number of occasions, and he was always nice, polite, and brilliant for a good sound bite. Even so, it's disconcerting when you see someone you think you know intimately and he turns out to be a celebrity instead. "Dr. Art Eulene!" I once heartily greeted the *Today* show's then-health correspondent on an airplane, believing he was my doctor, or perhaps my dentist. He smiled weakly and waved a tentative hand—I think he got that a lot.

Marc Jacobs was the only show I went to during the season a month after I had my first child. I was completely sleep deprived and barely fit my clothes, and I stumbled backstage feeling (and doubtless looking) like a zombie. But there was the champagne and the shiny hair and the cool, happy atmosphere—I felt almost like normal person. I had to interview the actual Marc Jacobs—something inane about how the makeup and hair reflected the spirit of his clothes—and while I never caught the much-hoped-for glimmer of recognition in his eyes (at last! my old friend!), I did feel vaguely, fashionably satisfied.

Sex and Fashion

I don't dream of *sleeping* with Marc Jacobs (though my friend Stella does, despite the fact that she's usually after a woman and he most definitely is not), but Tom Ford—unsurprisingly, to all who have seen or heard him—is an entirely different animal. He is gorgeous—both in a model-y, fashion-y way and in a rough, western-hero-guy way—and brilliant, magnetic, etc., etc. When he launched his first fragrance for Gucci, the aptly named Rush, I got an invitation to what I assumed was a typical big song-and-dance fragrance launch at the Carlyle. Once there, I was directed up to a private guest room, which seemed a little strange (you'd think you'd meet in the lobby perhaps, or the restaurant, it being a business meeting), but I went with it.

I opened the door to a beautiful, expansive suite with a gorgeous view of the park and no one in it—except, I soon saw, Tom Ford, *sitting on the bed.* He motioned for me to sit down *next to him on the bed,* and for the next forty or so minutes we discussed—he in his soft, gravelly, sexy voice—what sorts of things he found sexy or, as he put it, gave him "a rush." They were all sexually ambiguous remembrances from high school, lots of Santa Fe and hot sun and pools and pot smoking.

Tom Ford also has the incredible ability to talk about himself in a way that makes it seem that somehow he's listening to you rather than the other way around. Many designers have this same odd sort of charm, where you think one thing is happening in your conversation, when in fact it's just the opposite. Spend an evening with Michael Kors and you'll think you yourself are a very funny person. You not only believe you've been contributing wittily to the uproarious conversation all evening, you also believe you know lots about the real Michael Kors. But really, you've been sitting there mesmerized, your mouth hanging open like a fish, gasping for air between laughs. You know as much about Michael Kors personally as you know about Chris Rock after his *Comedy Central* special.

In the case of Tom Ford, the strategy involves sex, sex, and more sex appeal, and it works. Needless to say, when he finally unveiled the fragrance, I would've plastered it on the cover of *Elle*, would that I could.

Plus, I (and I'm sure every other woman who meets him) fully understand that he's gay, but the thing is, after the sexy-voiced, superpersonal-but-not "rush" stories, we just don't care.

Of course, when he quit fashion and subsequently rushed headlong back into beauty, everyone was in a whirl. A reporter grilled me (and, it turned out, every other beauty editor) for what felt like two hours—I had about seven million kids in my car, all of them screaming and fighting in the backseat as I calmly formulated answer after answer—on what I thought the new Tom Ford for Estée Lauder beauty line would be like: the packaging, the products, the scent . . . "If I knew, I'd be rich, because I'd have already made it myself!" I finally blurted rudely.

"If Tom Ford made you a lip gloss, what would it be called?" *Sex.*

"If Tom Ford created a new fragrance, what would it be called?" *Sex, Sex, and More Sex.*

"If Tom Ford wrote a memoir, what would it be called?" *How and Why I Gave Up Homosexuality for Jean Godfrey-June.* Anyway.

Chanel

Mansions are fabulous, and scores of mansions dotted around the globe are even more fabulous, but a compound is where it's at. Think Hyannis Port; think Agnelli-and-gardens; think rue Cambon, where the Chanel glamour industrial complex/compound resides, which I got to see once on a press trip to Paris. First, there's the string of shops along the Cambon cobblestones; upstairs is Coco Chanel's apartment, preserved as if in amber with giant crystal pears drooping from the chandeliers like sap from an enormous tropical tree and an apartment-size beige suede sofa quilted just like one of the famous bags.

High above that there's the Chanel version of a sweatshop: an airy, top-of-the-building atelier packed with gorgeous aging Frenchwomen (and their tiny, yapping dogs) who stitch each glittering couture paillette by hand. It looks like more women are at work than there really are, because the long tables are punctuated with hulking gray dress forms wrapped with rolls and rolls of heavy wool, so as to approximate the true figures of the women purchasing the couture (proof at last that most people who are too rich are actually *not* too thin). Each form has a name tag pinned to its chest on a little piece of paper, like undershirts in the laundry at a girls' school: Mme. X., super-rich person; Mme. Y., reigning political wife; Mme. Z., famous socialite. (No photographs! our guides hastened to add as we filed into the room, as we all imagined what fun the *New York Post* could be having with such a picture.)

The forms oddly reflected the figures of the women working on them (normal, middle-aged women) rather than those of the supermodels you'd expect to see wearing them; there was something sweet and tender, almost affectionate, going on between the sewing women and their forms. The warm afternoon breeze wafted across the room like a balm. Perhaps you get—along with the tiny hand stitches and the supposed revolutionary thinking that the magazines swoon over when they run their many pieces on the couture that 1/89 millionth of their readers can afford—a garment infused with some kindness, some good intention, that's lacking in our otherwise hard-edged, off-the-rack world.

Either way, it doesn't come cheap. Deep in the bowels of the same building, in marble corridors than run under the street, they showed us the Chanel archives, filled with all sorts of beautiful items, the most dumbfounding of which was a dress—one of three identical ones bought for three glamorous sisters by their mother—gorgeous and beaded and all, that cost roughly $230,000 apiece.

That night, we had dinner in an enormous ballroom festooned with red silk curtains, unbelievably beautiful flowers, crystal goblets of champagne . . . we watched the sun set over the Ritz, looked out through the ancient French doors over the Place de la Concorde, and reflected upon our incredible good luck (or most of us did, anyway). I was even luckier and got to sit at the table of Chanel's worldwide president, Mme. F. (that's *F* for *français*).

The conversation, given the surroundings, naturally turned to love. One of my fellow American beauty editors began telling us the story of how she met her husband. "Well," she began, "I wasn't getting any younger." Mme. F. looked a little shocked. "So I decided to get mathematical about it." We all leaned in. "I drew up a list of every single man I knew of, in alphabetical order, and I just started going down the list!" Mme. F. was now visibly blanching a bit. "I went on one date with each man, and on each date, I asked him point-blank: 'Could you see yourself getting married within the next year or two?' Naturally, my husband's name starts with Z!"

We thought that was it, and that somehow the visibly

distressed Mme. F. was going to recover, but the editor kept on. "So we started dating, and after a few months, I told him I wanted to get engaged within the next four months. He said okay." At that moment, the chasm between France and America seemed wider than a nation's worth of Wal-Marts.

"At the end of the four months, I woke him up bright and early. 'Today's the day, honey!' I said. So we got engaged! And we've been married two years now!" Mme. F. tried gamely to join the conversations that followed that evening, managing to repress the French blood that doubtless boiled in her veins, wanting nothing more than to sputter her incredulous dismay; and I have to say, for once, I felt a French person's pain.

Chanel and My Personal Designer-Label Inoculation Program

I learned an important fashion lesson from Chanel. A beauty product with the Chanel label on it, more than any other—Gucci, Marc Jacobs, Armani, whatever—is the closest thing in the cosmetics industry to a fistful of cash. If you offer a person with horribly dry skin a Chanel toner formulated for the oily and acne prone, she'll snap it up in a millisecond, take it home, and prop it up in her bathroom, never to be used except to radiate its proud, iconic glamour. Those two C's confer a value on objects—from a tiny base coat for your nails to enormous handbags—that's truly astounding, absolutely unwavering, and hard not to buy into. For a long time, all I wanted was Chanel, Chanel, Chanel, and of course, I couldn't afford it.

There's nothing on earth like the Chanel sample sale, which happens twice a year and reminds me, in its unwavering set of traditions year to year, of university commencement exercises more than anything else. The sale is traditionally held in the ballroom of a fading-but-still-on-Central-Park-West hotel. It opens at 8:00 a.m.; editors—editors in chief, fashion editors, and beauty editors—plus a smattering of publishers begin lining up around 7:00 a.m. Cutting in line can be a reflection of incredible power or incredible naïveté.

The feeling is, if you're there, you've sort of made it. And everyone who's anyone sees you there, so they know you've made it. The floodgates are opened, and everyone rushes for the merch, then rips off their clothes in front of everyone to try everything on, laughing and shrieking the whole time as if they're at some big sorority sleepover party. I always got things—and though it's a sample sale, it's Chanel, so it's not exactly dirt cheap: $200 for once-$500 shoes, that sort of thing—that had the two C's but, like the acne toner for the dry skin person, were never quite me.

The year I had my daughter, India, I got a lot of presents from a pricey department store, most of which I returned (how many baby rattles can one child actually rattle?) for store credit. The credit had to be used by the end of the year. At the same time, I hadn't seen the shows, hadn't looked at magazines, even for that season, so everything in the stores looked ugly and confusing to me. "How am I going to use up this credit?" I wailed to my wily, brilliant friend Jennifer.

"Get a Chanel jacket," she said firmly. "Even if you don't wear it right now, you'll wear it till you're eighty."

So I did.

I marched in and bought, full-price, the iconic navy blue Chanel jacket—and I've never gone to another sample sale. Sometimes if you get the über-thing, the thing that never goes on sale that they're using as a carrot to sell you all the other stuff, you can save yourself a lot of money, time, and clutter.

Victoria's Secret

The Victoria's Secret show is like any other fashion show except that it's not a fashion show at all, it's a *show* show. Closer to *Cabaret* than Miu Miu. The underwear that minces down the runway is not always for sale (not that regular runway shows don't feature purely "editorial," not-for-actual-purchase shock-and-awe items, but Victoria's Secret, with its million-dollar diamond-studded bras and the beribboned angels' wings it mounts on the backs of the models, takes this license to its logical extreme).

Instead of fashion editors and retailers, the stands are filled with lingerie editors, beauty editors, and male celebs who come to drool. From Tommy Lee to Magic Johnson to Woody Harrelson to the odd stockbroker with a really excellent fashion connection, the men sit, wide legged as if they owned the place, smirking out at the runway as if it contained their personal harem, from which they might select a companion for the evening. If cigars were allowed, they'd all be sucking suggestively on them.

Gisele and co. flounce out in tiny nothings made to seem all the tinier by the huge prosthetic *Angels in America* wings they wear. There are sideshows—flying trapeze artists in shiny white-nylon sausage-casing suits overhead, Oscar-half-time-appropriate duets with Mary J. Blige and Sting—with TV cameras set perfectly in place to get the best angle. Cirque du Soleil is supposedly always on the hunt for new themes for their bazillion-dollar permanent shows in Vegas, and I can't believe they've ignored Victoria's Secret for as long as they have, because everyone involved would make an enormous amount of money.

The security is legendary; fur protesters are always lying in wait, despite the fact that Victoria's Secret doesn't sell fur. Models sell fur, goes the reasoning, and since the cameras are trained on them at this show more than any other, this is the place to protest. No matter what your feelings on the subject of fur, however, it seems (as it happened one year) more than mean—almost downright evil—to attack a woman who's standing there in her underwear with enormous wings attached to her back in front of millions of people. It seems stupid, actually, because you end up drumming up sympathy for the model, not your cause.

Secret Ingredient

There's a designer famous in Euro circles for a rather disturbing predilection for excrement. We all have our peccadillos. I hadn't really thought about it much until I was sitting in the presentation for his newest fragrance, which I loved: It was the cleanest, best, nicest scent, and he had specially designed it so, though subtle, it would last all day long. Subtle fragrances always last for about two seconds; you usually have to wear a really over-the-top one if you want it to last all day. So—brilliant! I was sold! I'd be wearing it every day! But then the presenter started talking about, as he put it, "the coup de grâce," "the thing that makes this fragrance different from any other," "a secret, sensual ingredient" that the designer had insisted upon to "make it sexy." "None of us even knows what this ingredient, this note, might be," continued the presenter. "All we know is it is very *sensual* for him."

Fashion Shows

As I've intimated with the Marc Jacobs experiences, fashion shows are one of the most entertaining things on earth: the hottest girls on the planet in usually at least nominally sexy outfits, marching and swinging to concert-decible music mixed by the hottest DJs on the planet. The front rows are splattered with crazy celebs (my favorites are the ones who take notes studiously, as if they're taking in an important lecture on Kant), socialites, and, most glamorous to me, the magazine people with their studied "thrown on" outfits and their elaborate pecking order that's subtly adjusted from show to show via the seating arrangements.

Backstage, while it sounds wildly glamorous and rock-concert-y, is generally a big bore; everyone, from the designer and the models to the makeup artists and stylists to the hair assistants, thinks they're a great big star doing very important work (magazine and TV types are back there documenting it all in stultifying detail, so who can blame them?), and everyone's very stressed out and do-you know-who-I-*am*?

Beauty editors are always sent backstage to "get the story" direct from the makeup artists and hairstylists as they're creating the looks. It's often staged and uncomfortable, but it can also be exciting and creative and real. It can also be trouble.

The Chanel show in Paris is always held at the crack of dawn on the last day of the shows, so everyone's a little cranky along with their usual self-importance and stress-fueled intolerance. One year I was backstage, exhausted, furiously taking notes backstage: "Barrette on far side of head." "Use spray." "Pale pink gloss, black liner." Thrilling stuff. Kate Moss (whom I will always worship as the most beautiful woman ever to exist, no matter what people say) and Amber Valletta sat in the chairs in front of me as a team of hairdressers worked on them. "Kate straight, Amber gets hair cream, very 1920s."

"YOU," snarled Amber, pointing a *j'accuse* index finger at me. Kate, my beloved idol, whirled around to look at me in horror. "What are you writing about?" Amber demanded.

"I—I'm the beauty editor from *Elle*," I stammered.

"I don't care who you are, you can't invade our privacy!"

"I'm taking notes on your hair."

"Whatever." They turned, flipping their fabulous hair with the disgust that only the most popular girls can properly dish out.

But once the lights go up, the music starts blasting, and models appear in full work-it mode, who cares? It's a thrill few people can resist. You're on the inside, and you're getting to watch this incredible show that only a select few will ever see live. Men always act as if a fashion show is the dullest thing they can imagine; I once snuck the intrepid Gary into a Todd Oldham show back when Cindy and Naomi and co., with their amazing bodies and their faces that didn't challenge anyone's notions about conventional beauty, were in full force—and he instantly gained about 50 percent more respect for my career.

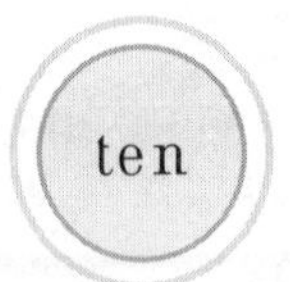

The Haircut That Changed My Life

No name impresses a celebrity—designer or otherwise—more than "Sally." You've got your Tom, your Julia, your Brad, and your Angelina . . . they all pale before Sally. Sally is a hairdresser, and nothing impresses her.

The myth is (and it remains a myth because I'm far too frightened to ask) that Sally is fantastically, independently wealthy, and that's why she doesn't care. But if fantastic independent wealth were all it took to be Sally, there'd be nobody left to do unseemly reality shows or make asses out of themselves at the country club. Sally is (seemingly) effortlessly slim, beautiful, cool, and on top of things. She won't cut your hair for less than $600, and she won't do it anyway because the waiting list is six trillion years long.

Just the way Crème de la Mer started the trend for astronomically expensive skin creams—the price itself somehow a testament to the power of the cream inside—so Sally started the trend for astronomically expensive haircuts. Just like Crème de la Mer, she's quickly been outpriced by competitors, and just like Crème de la Mer, she remains the original.

If you've got the $600 and you make it past the six tril-

Is Crème de la Mer Worth It?

A dear friend (thankfully now in perfect health) had breast cancer and thus had to have radiation. I didn't know this, but whatever part of your body gets the radiation ends up with radiation burns—along with incredibly irritated, roughed-up skin all around. They give you a special ointment to put on it but tell you to prepare for the worst anyway.

This friend of mine, ever glamorous, substituted Crème de la Mer. When the treatments were finished and she went for a checkup with the oncologist, his jaw dropped in amazement when he examined the spot where the burn should have been. "I've never seen anything like this in my entire career!" he blurted. "This is incredible!" Then, of course, he had to know what cream she was using.

- They also tell you, the second you're diagnosed with breast cancer, to quit using antiperspirant. Magazines are forever trumpeting the lack of evidence linking breast cancer and antiperspirants, but when you actually get it, the doctors tell another story.
- Crème de la Mer is genius on other burns as well. Do the cold thing—ice, ice, ice, until you can stand it no more—and then slather on the La Mer. Why not feel glamorous when you're wincing in pain, after all? A spoonful of sugar and all that.

lion years, you've got Sally to contend with. She takes herself utterly seriously. She considers every client with an unflinching gaze; you get the feeling that if you said something that turned out to be uncool, she might turn away, drop her scissors in a relaxed sort of disgust, and simply walk away. So you don't say much.

Sally's delicate features belie an absolutely unshakable sense of conviction. If you're on a shoot with her, and if the photographer isn't either Annie Leibowitz or Steven Meisel, she'll give him or her very pointed, direct advice on camera angles and lighting techniques. She's got plenty to say to the makeup people and the fashion editors as well. She directs her assistants with a style straight out of *Apocalypse Now.*

She's tiny, and her outfit is always the same: jeans, Birkenstocks, a Petit Bateau T-shirt. She claims to shop furiously at places like Gucci, but the only evidence of it is the occasional tough-girl leather cuff on one arm. Sally's favorite word is *major,* as in, "Your hair's going to be *major,*" or, "That girl is just so *major.*"

Her hair is always the same: early Mia Farrow meets early Jane Fonda (the shag period). Sally is famous for having cut Meg Ryan's tousled *When Harry Met Sally/You've Got Mail* shag; some people like to say she always gives people that same haircut, which can't be, as she cuts everyone's hair in Hollywood, and they don't all have cute shags.

Her salon in Los Angeles is built around a shallow turquoise swimming pool: Glass walls on all sides look in on it and across at one another. It's very Hollywood, very gossipy, very secret affair. The one in New York is a huge meatpacking district loft that floats above the Stella McCartney store. The two art pieces that dominate the New York one encapsulate Sally's take-no-prisoners, be-yourself-and-kick-major-ass approach to beauty for me: When you walk in, there's an enormous black-and-white Bert Stern of Marilyn Monroe—the famous final shoot—that Marilyn herself slashed a big, antiglamour X across. A few paces past, in the main salon, is a wall-size, deep crimson lithograph of the very young Jane Fonda's mug shot—tough, shaggy, natural, impossibly beautiful. Even the fanciest girly-girl socialite couldn't resist wanting to be Jane Fonda in that picture.

But the decor is not the point (though it sets you into a dreamy state of hope and anticipation). Every good hairstylist's biggest talent is the ability to direct their attention fully on another person, to take in whoever they're looking at, and to make that person feel seen and carefully considered. Sally, for me, goes a step further and has no agenda about how she wants her clients to look. They don't all have to be polished, or rough, or sexy, or uptown-y or downtown-y. You don't look at people and instantly know Sally cut their hair.

Sally will tell you the truth, no matter who you are: I think that's why the celebs all love her—the last thing they need is another yes-man.

She once threw me out. I arrived at her meatpacking district salon, sat amid the pictures and filled with hope and anticipation. But she shook her head when she saw me. "No," she said. "Your hair's good right now. Come back in about three weeks. You guys"—she gestured to her trembling assistants (always hot, always underground-y, always male)—"isn't her hair good right now? Like, I don't think we should cut it. No."

I was once in Sally's chair when Courtney Love blazed in. Tough and Tougher. "Sally," she said, "you're going to do my hair for this weird indie movie in New Jersey in a few weeks, and then you'll do it a couple months later for this big-budget one, tons of money. Okay?"

Sally studied her. She put her hands on her hips. She frowned. At last she breathed. "Courtney," she said. "Honey? No. We need to do something *now.*"

All I know is, it's pointless to drop your famous friend X. or Y.—even your superfamous friend X. or Y.—with most people.

Who cares, at the end of the day, if you've had dinner with Renée Zellweger? But if you're trying to impress Renée herself—or her agent, or a huge producer, or a huge director—just casually drop in a little Sally reference. The beauty angle trumps everything in Hollywood, and there is no other Sally.

I Went to L.A. and All I Got Were These Lousy Implants!

I come from a generally less-well-endowed family (except for one relative who had a small reduction to get rid of back pain, etc., and was generally pleased) and am personally the size that, had I decided to be an actress in Hollywood, I might feel pressure to get a boob job.

Here's my trouble with all movie stars' biggest obsession: Grandma Helen, a wise, almost shamanistic figure for me, always warned me strenuously that when you get old (old as in seventy) your breasts get much, much larger, and, as she put it, "it's no fun."

When the Wonderbra first came out, I was sent a very aggressive one, and I tried it out one day. I got much, much more male attention than usual, but the males who were paying attention to me were uniformly either construction workers or homeless people.

Not that I don't appreciate the sexifying and slimmifying (they throw everything into a slightly different proportion) effects of slightly larger breasts, which I experienced while breast-feeding. (Why everyone in Hollywood doesn't simply breast-feed for all eternity—it makes you both skinny and well endowed—is beyond me.)

In Los Angeles, I delight my friends by divining which women have had implants. I'm almost always right. There's a shelf quality to most of them that's hard to escape.

The first time I went to Sally, she looked at me for a minute and sent me in for the shampoo. Until then, I'd always blown my hair dry—not to make it straight, just to make it look, I thought, better. I emerged from the shampoo room with my wet, wavy hair dripping around my shoulders. She considered me again. "You've got this Gisele thing happening," she said. "You've got to throw out your blow dryer and never use it again." She circled around me a third time and harrumphed in a triumphant sort of way. "And no more bangs, and for the real Gisele, you need a middle part."

Someday they'll discover the reason for the "grass is always greener" impulse. Most people have major "grass is greener" issues surrounding their hair—if it's straight, they want waves and volume; if it's curly, they want it flat and straight; if it's brown, they want blond, and then they want red. . . . I'm lucky to have escaped it, except that all the "grass is always greener" insecurity was simply transferred into another category—skin color, which is crazier, if you think about it. You

You can find a gorgeous model who has your hair.

You can. This is the lesson of Sally.

I'd been a bangs-wearing, side-part blow-dryer girl since I'd triumphed over my mother and grown out my pixie, and I was unwilling to change it until Sally brought up Gisele. Until I quit blow-drying my hair, no one but hairstylists told me what great hair I had. Post Sally, post blow dryer, everyone does.

color your hair only every month or two—self-tanner, on the other hand, lasts about three days.

The Sally lesson, as noted, is that most people are prettiest with some not-too-modified version of their natural hair texture. One of my roommates in college blew her hair straight every day, even if she was going out for a jog. She forbade all of us to use her car, but one rainy night she called us from the library. "*My keys are on my nightstand!*" she stage-whispered into the phone. "*Get over here right now!* And drive right up on the lawn! I'll pay the ticket!" The rain, she explained, would make her hair curl, and even though it was pitch black outside and we were all of three blocks away, someone might see her.

A few months later, there was a party where everyone (including the roommate) got thrown in the pool. She'd drunk enough that she didn't care—and none of us could believe how gorgeous she suddenly looked. Including the boy she'd had a crush on for the previous two years, who asked her out the next day.

My own self-acceptance in the hair department may have something to do with my forced-pixie childhood, not to mention the fact that my hair was always fairly straight until I had a baby (I know this is an old wives' tale that's physically impossible, but it definitely happened, possible or not). So all my life I longed for long, wavy hair, and now I have it. But, of course, it's all wrong unless I'm tan tan tan.

It can also go all wrong anyway; even with the self-acceptance, I must note, there is no escape from the bad hair day—days where I wake, Kafka-like, to find myself resembling either Bill Clinton or Naomi Wolf. Bill Clinton is a handsome man, and Naomi Wolf is a beautiful woman, but my looking like either of them is not pretty at all. I know it's just hair, but that's the thing about a bad hair day—it takes over and infects your entire being, moving quickly from your hair to your skin to your expression to your entire demeanor.

As far as I can tell, I get the Clinton when my hair's too puffy and the Wolf when it's too straight, but the parameters, in reality, are not so clear. I can brush, I can rearrange, I can run styling cream through the ends, but the only cure for a Clinton/Wolf is to take a shower and wash it all out.

I once had a Donald Trump day, which was truly the worst; I hope never to repeat it, but there—it did happen.

The Look

The look is everything when it comes to the world of fancy, high-priced hairstylists. I don't mean the look that a particular stylist gives your hair, I mean the way they look at you and how that look makes you feel special. The look is also the reason for the frequency with which homely-looking photographers end up with fantastically gorgeous models: Like a hairdresser, someone who's taking your picture is really, really paying you some attention. Leos are always described as having huge manes; my theory is there's a little bit of Leo in everyone, and it all comes out when you're talking about hair. (More re astrology and hair later on.)

For one of my first articles at *Elle,* I had to trail Mark Garrison, a top stylist at Frederic Fekkai (and now an owner of his own glamorous Madison Avenue salon, P.S.), for a day in the salon. Client after client sat down in his chair, only to have him rouse them back out of it so they could stand in front of him so he could see how their hair fell. There they'd stand, nervous and hopeful, and invariably he'd point out—disguised in the discussion of what they wanted to do with their hair—how stunningly gorgeous one or more of their features were. The people were not stunningly gorgeous, but everything he said about them was true. One had beautiful skin, another had striking gray eyes, another great bone structure.

"How do you keep your hair so shiny?" he asked the unenthusiastic (she'd been scheduled to see Fekkai, but he was out sick; she'd asked her husband how short he thought she should go and he'd shrugged disinterestedly), overweight, fifty-something woman from St. Barts.

"I wear a hat," she said, lighting up like a Christmas tree, unaware of her apathetic companion and exuding calm and grace.

When it was the bored husband's turn to stand before Garrison, he got a "Is this *all* your natural color?" and an "Incredible hair." The man stood taller and puffed out his chest, nodding agreeably. The couple left the salon holding hands, clearly happy and not the slightest bit perturbed that they'd missed out on seeing their regular stylist.

Shake Your Hair, Darling

"It's nice to be complimented," said Garrison when I asked him about it. "No one hears it enough." He went on to say that there was "always" a sexual dynamic with every client, male or female (Garrison had a girlfriend at the time). He had every client shake their hair for him as they stood there. "They're participating," he said. "I see what their hair is doing, but it helps them get into it, feel my focus on them."

Trixie

My friend Jennifer is a gorgeous girl and has always attracted throngs of handsome men, but back in our days of several-parties-per-night-no-exceptions, we observed an admittedly anecdotal but astonishingly powerful phenomenon: On a lark, Jennifer purchased a cheap blond hairpiece (she is blond)—the kind you stab in at the top of your hair and it makes you look as if you've got lots more volume than you really do. Understand: This hairpiece didn't change the color or length of her hair in any way. It just added a little volume. She called it Trixie. She put Trixie in one night before we went to a party. *Every* man loved her. Not some, not most, *all*. She tried it again the next night. And again. With Trixie in her hair, she attracted at least 30 percent more men, without fail.

Something to think about before you spend all that money on a boob job or whatever.

Once, when I was freelancing for *Seventeen*, we brought a model to have her hair cut for the cameras by a hugely important stylist whose private cutting room had six chairs, all of them filled with eager clients—that day, several big socialites, a famous model, and our model, whom we'd dressed in a Chanel ball gown. A wildly glamorous scene. The stylist's drug problem, we soon discovered, had advanced to a point where he remembered only the focusing-on-the-client part. He buzzed officiously from chair to chair, touching hair, exclaiming over the beauty of each woman, appraising, nodding. He'd disappear after a few minutes into the back with his assistant, emerge giggling and trailing french fries, and do the circuit again. "It's perfect!" he at last announced to the famous model. "I love it! You look fantastic."

"But X.," said the model, aghast, "you haven't done anything to it."

He stared at her, not comprehending what she was saying.

"You're supposed to *cut* my hair."

Indeed, the (usually drug-related) perils of being so incredibly talented at people pleasing are significant. I'm sure if they compared the number of drug addicts in hairdressing with that in almost any other profession, they'd top the list. There was one stylist, Didier Martheleur, who was on his way up when I was first freelancing at *Vogue*. We all loved him—he was charming and confident and talented and made everyone feel beautiful and unique. He made piles of money, went out with piles of beautiful models, and got his own salon at the tender age of nineteen. Two years later he died of an overdose, leaving behind a gorgeous model wife and a four-year-old.

I wish the attention-lavishing talent could be cultivated or bottled; it would make someone very rich. Fountain-of-youth rich, I think: You can have anyone you want if you can look at people with your full attention, I'm convinced—no matter what you look like. Some large portion of inner beauty involves the ability to see the beauty in others and really focus in on it.

I try: If I notice something I like about someone—their shirt or their hair or their skin, whatever—I say so. But so far, no one's fallen at my feet and begged me to sleep with them.

You Can't Have Everything

I went to a glamorous art world party. Everyone was mind-bendingly rich and ironic. Thrilled and horrified by the fabulousness swirling around me, I cast about desperately for a conversation not about buying vast tracts of land upstate. In the corner by the champagne, I met a man who was talking earnestly and unironically about astrology. "It's just my hobby," I overheard him explaining to several assembled *artistes.* "Like you," he said pointing straight at me as if in sudden recognition. "You have Leo hair and a Cancer face."

It's true: I am indeed on the cusp of Leo and Cancer; further, my hair is indeed much more fabulous than my face.

I've always thought of myself as a Leo, perhaps in denial over the shy, more watery aspects of my personality (not all Cancers are shy and watery, but sweeping generalizations and ugly stereotypes are rarely permitted in any context anywhere nowadays, so I relish the chance to air them when I get the chance).

Adam, whose birthday falls two days after mine, characterizes the Leo/Cancer cusp dweller as a "reluctant diva," a description that fits us both quite well. He has spent a large part of our friendship pointing out the discrepancies in magazine astrology columns; depending on the magazine, my birthday oscillates between Cancer and Leo. "I don't think you're a Leo at all," he'll say, peering at *Vogue,* which has me as a Cancer. I snap back at him with a *Allure,* where I'm a day into Leo.

In any case, this stranger had come to the truth of it: Leo hair and a Cancer face. At the very least, this gives a good dimestore psychology reason for my long enchantment with self-tanner—an attempt to compensate for my deeply un-Leo unsunniness, perhaps.

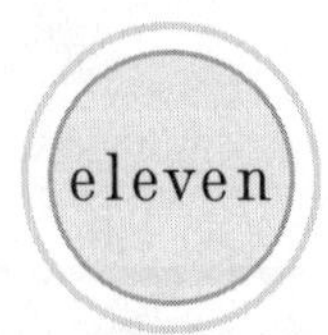

Inner Beauty; or, What I Learned at the Spa

My original spa experiences were with my high school/collegiate constant companion, Julia. Julia's parents were modern people in ways that most of the parents weren't: Her father ran the psychology department at Stanford, and her mother taught assertiveness training and she taught it in no small way, writing bestselling books and running workshops at places like Hewlett-Packard and IBM. They talked about things—sex, condoms, interpersonal relationships as if they were no big deal, which greatly impressed me. A small Picasso nude hung over their king-size bed. Their home was constantly being redecorated in ever-more-sophisticated shades of beige. Julia's parents had it going on.

In their usual groundbreaking way, Julia's parents joined a gym. This was before there were gyms, really; people had just started to jog in California. It wasn't even called a gym—it was called a spa. "Gotta go to the spa," they'd say, rushing out the door, towels slung perfectly over their shoulders. It seemed deeply glamorous.

One rainy day both Julia and I fell ill with a bad cold. Of

course, we called each other. Julia had a brilliant idea: "They have a hot tub at the spa," she said. "Wouldn't it feel great to breathe in all that warm air, and soak in the warm water?" We rolled up towels, swung them over our shoulders, stole her mother's I.D., snuck in, and spent over half a day in that hot tub, turning to shriveled prunes and doubtlessly infecting countless spa patrons with our noxious colds. We were deliriously happy, and very relaxed. There's just something about a spa, especially the going-to-a-spa-with-a-girlfriend, that makes even a lone hot tub in a health club full of Thighmasters feel like a special and memorable occasion.

Our next spa adventure occurred in Istanbul, Turkey, during college. We'd flown to Turkey from Greece (lest we sound more fabulous than we were, the flight cost $20 and we were met by a line of Turkish troops that pointed their bayonettes at us as we inched gingerly off the plane to collect our scrappy "Let's Go!" backpacks). It was sunny in Greece when we left and pouring rain in Istanbul when we arrived. Julia, who had blond hair that reached past her waist, happened to be wearing a hot-pink minidress—perfect for the beach in Greece, not so perfect for the streets of Istanbul, teeming as they were with staunchly Islamic men.

No women were to be seen anywhere that day, so the mere fact of our presence caused a stir, never mind the blonde hair and the pink minidress in the pouring rain. Despite this, we had to find the youth hostel, so there was nothing to do but walk the streets (parallel intentional) until we found it.

Julia, always more open-minded and friendly than I've ever managed to be, was, throughout our European sojourn, far more interested than I in cultural exchange. Obviously lecherous men would approach in cafés and at train stations, and she would eagerly engage them in conversation, thrilled to practice the language, get an insider track on what to see, etc. She was always shocked anew, every time, when they became angry after she refused to go home with them.

So we walked down the wet streets of Istanbul, she smiling innocently and returning the many greetings we were receiving from strangers, me growing more and more strident as I fought the admirers off. The admirers became more insistent; they formed a pied-piper-like line down the street, clamoring for the attention of Julia. All at once, both of us panicked. We needed to get out of there. And suddenly, in front of us, a door, with stained glass shapes cut into it, and a sign that said "LADIES ENTRANCE." In we went, breathless and soaked to the bone.

It turned out to be a famous Turkish bath. We were thrilled. We showered and went to wait for the treatment in a huge, church-dome-like *hammam* full of steam. We lay on the huge marble benches, staring up as the clouds of steam wafted through the arc of the dome, up toward the tiny stained-glass stars and moon punched in the ancient ceiling. No men. No rain. Only heavy, warm steam. Sublime doesn't begin to describe it.

A few minutes later, out came the masseuses: Large (sumo-wrestler-sized) old women, wearing nothing but enormous, waist-high black-lace underpants, each of them holding a large block of black-mud soap. They soaped us up. We looked across at one another and smiled. Heaven. Then, with a loud grunt, they began beating us with the soap—technically, what they were doing might be called an extremely vigorous massage—jabbing the corners of it full-force into and under, say, your collarbone. Their strength was truly unbelievable, even given their size. After a minute or two, there was nothing to do but laugh, so painful and unexpected was the "massage." We shrieked and laughed, alternately; the women ignored it all and continued to pummel us. It continued for an hour; there was something very *Midnight Express* about the whole experience. At the end, they blasted us with a hoseful of highly pressurized salt water—no picnic, either. But as we lay there, jellified on the marble slabs after they'd finally left, we did feel fantastic.

Luckily, when we emerged, the admirers had dispersed, and we did eventually find the hostel. Incredibly, days later, we had no bruises, though our stomach muscles still hurt from all the convulsive, panicked laughter.

Perhaps the ultimate perk of the beauty editor job is the free spa stays. I wish I'd taken more advantage of it before having kids, because when you've got no time, a spa stay is just not in your future, not ever. I did get one plum assignment, back when I was freelancing: *Town & Country* had me go, undercover, to three major spas, each for a week, back to back. Does going to a spa work? When I say that my body was perfect after those three weeks, I mean it was *perfect.*

The idea behind the story was what did you get at the superluxe spa versus the middle-of-the-road versus the hard-core budget option. The luxe option was Maine Chance, the hundred-or-so-year-old Elizabeth Arden spa in Arizona, which sadly closed a month or so after I went there (so I never got to write the article). We (all women, all of them much older than me, all of them curious to know what my husband did that I was able to afford to go to Maine Chance at such a tender age) stayed in unbelievably fabulous, two-story, old-Hollywood-style bungalows outfitted in comfy but expensive pale-floral slipcovers. The sheets were Porthault, the dishes the thinnest bone china with the palest flowers, the crystal Baccarat; there were even little monogrammed mats placed in precisely the spot where your feet would land when you slid out of bed each morning.

Your breakfast arrived on a tray with a handwritten (Tiffany stationery) schedule of the day's activities: "Wrap, 9:30 a.m.; Facial, 2:00 p.m.," etc. What most intrigued me was the entry "Broth, 11:00 a.m.," and then again "Broth, 3:30 p.m." Broth turned out to be actual broth—beef-marrow broth, perhaps?—dispensed in small paper cups around the pool at particular times. The women gathered in their big white bathrobes by the pool, expectant. "Broth, broth!" the attendants barked, rather the way a proctor at a girls' school might shout, "Choir practice!" or, "Pledge of Allegiance!" Very much like patients in a mental ward, we—in the big bathrobes—would shuffle into a line to receive the broth and then retire to a chaise longue to drink it. It was never stated precisely, the function of the broth; I took it to be strengthening, reviving.

Perhaps spas used to be where you went after a nervous breakdown; the coddling was so intense that I did feel like a patient being brought along gently, gradually built back up and made ready for the chilly and challenging outside world.

The slow and predictable schedule of exercise, treatment, exercise (never terribly intense), treatment, had a lulling quality that was very pleasant—except for the hot-wax treatment, which I'd taken to be a euphemism but was not. I'd gone for a run in the hot Arizona sun and ran back across the vast acreage of the spa when I realized I was late for my next treatment. Still sweating, I stripped and lay in the cocoonlike layers of towels and plastic wrap the attendant had prepared for me on the table. Then she literally poured buckets of hot wax onto my naked and already boiling-hot body. This alone was painful, but it became worse when she finished with the buckets of molten wax and rolled me up in it, tucking the towels and plastic wrap around me as if she were fashioning a very snug burrito, and left me there to "heat up." When I complained that I thought I was getting overheated, she nodded sympathetically and put a cool cloth over my eyes and forehead, which was about as useful as a Band-Aid after open heart surgery.

I tried to escape (she'd left the room and did not respond to my calls), rolling around on the table, but I was completely immobilized and had to wait many torturous minutes before she finally arrived with another cold compress and I somehow managed to convince her to let me out.

You dressed for dinner at Maine Chance; there was silk and more silk and pink-wool skirt suits and lemon-yellow pantsuits and cocktail rings the size of jawbreakers. They had models walk through in Escada and St. John ensembles that cost thousands of dollars. The ladies—bright eyed at last after the long day of sumptuous lethargy, their hair coiffed and their makeup perfect—scribbled the numbers of the outfits they wanted and passed them to the attendants. "What does your husband do again?" they kept demanding, clearly perplexed. I wasn't ready for Escada or St. John. But even with the obvious not belonging and the less-than-invigorating pace, if Maine Chance were still in existence, I'd urge every woman I know to go there. In terms of relaxation—and I've seen more than my share of theories about the best ways to relax—there's nothing like being a rich mental patient for a week. Nothing.

Number two was the hard-core budget spa the Ashram, up in

the hills near Los Angeles. They starve you at the Ashram, and they work you to death, everyone said. And you have to share a room. To make the article funny, I stopped outside a Longs drugstore on my way there, bought a package of peanut-butter-fudge Girl Scout cookies, and tucked them into my bag. Contraband.

The Ashram resides in a split-level 1970s L.A. ranch house, and not a very nice one at that. "Unassuming" is the kindest way I can put it: faded-out sheets, peeling paint, lots of chipped Formica. I had gone the cheapest route possible, which was to sleep on the porch—and the porch, with the world outside all around, actually seemed more luxurious than the rooms.

There were three bathrooms for twelve guests to share, a serious problem given the fact that we were permitted no caffeine and barely any food—so everyone became constipated almost immediately. There was a single, very public (directly adjacent to one of the bathrooms) pay phone. I think the idea was sort of a love-your-neighbor bonding experience, but for me (and many of my compatriots) it was much more a hell-is-other-people-if-I-have-to-look-at-you-for-one-more-second-I'll-scream sort of thing.

They woke you up in the morning, and you did several hours of yoga in a little yurt before breakfast. Breakfast was either an orange or a glass of orange juice. I had signed up for "extra food" since I didn't need to lose much weight at the time, so I and several others received a piece of melba toast as well. Then it was out into the hot L.A. canyons for a many-hour, very strenuous hike.

The front-runners on each hike were the saddest people who exist on our earth: Hollywood wives. This one was that producer's wife, that one was married to a famous actor. They were the sweetest, friendliest, nicest women, they were good-

Spa Lessons

Over the course of my career, I've visited a number of spas—from one in St. Lucia called Le Sport to Canyon Ranch in the Berkshires—and I've learned several important things:

1. Spas aimed at Europeans are never going to make you skinny. You will be drunk, fat, and relaxed.

2. Never get a salt scrub after sitting out in the sun for any length of time whatsoever.

3. Three is always a crowd. Don't visit a spa with more than one extra friend or less than four; someone will be killed or at least not get a chance to relax.

4. Hydrotherapy cellulite treatments consist of being lined up, execution-style, against a wall and being blasted with a hose fit for a fire hydrant. They hurt, and you feel vaguely violated afterward.

5. Spas spend all their money on the big, public spaces they can picture in their brochures. The rooms are never good (since Maine Chance has closed, anyway), so adjust your expectations accordingly.

6. You can eat as much as you like of low-calorie, soft-serve ice-cream substitutes; you will never be satisfied.

looking as hell, but they were desperate. Instead of walking (which was effort enough, even for the instructors), the poor Hollywood wives jogged ahead, intent on burning as many calories as humanly possible, on getting that much more tone into their muscles. They (there were three; none of them knew one another before they came to the Ashram, but they were instant companions, if only because they were so far ahead of everyone else) scurried along no matter how hot it got, always looking as if they were about to cry. At the end of the line was a woman from Long Island who was deep, deep into Kundalini yoga, and she groaned loudly as she hiked along slowly, her cries echoing in the hills. At times it sounded as if she were in pain, at times as if she were having an especially satisfying orgasm.

The rest of us, in the middle, suffered along. There was a crazy older man who said that he came to the Ashram four times a year (you're not allowed to go consecutive weeks) and that he drank and ate wildly in between. There was the woman we all wanted to kill who talked only of herself, her body and her discontents with it, and her many expensive possessions back home. There was a screenwriter whose wife had sent him there for his fortieth birthday and a book editor about my age (my roommate on the porch), among others.

After the death-defying hike, there was "lunch," either a small bowl of lentil soup or a lentil-and-sprout salad, each option unbelievably tiny.

Then you'd do some sort of exercise in the overalgaed pool or get the one luxury you got each day: a really good, hour-long massage from one of the handsomest men you'll ever see, outdoors, with the Pachelbel Canon playing. It was fantastic unless the Kundalini lady happened to be getting her massage at the same time, in which case you were treated to her anguished/orgasmlike cries throughout.

Then there was a second, late-afternoon hike, several more hours of yoga, and a few lentils for dinner. Afterward they lectured us on a breed of people they claimed existed called the

Breath-Airians (Breath Aryans?) who exist solely on air and wander various forests in South America, perfectly healthy without any form of nourishment at all save a very focused ability to meditate. The lectures quickly sent us all into a stupor.

On the last night, after "dinner," I whispered my secret—the Girl Scout cookies, which lay untouched at the bottom of my bag—to the two people I could actually stand, the screenwriter and my roommate on the porch, the book editor. Though I have one of the heartiest appetites of any woman I know (I eat more than anyone, including my husband and many male friends; my mother is the only person who can beat me, really, and it's just unbelievable luck that I'm not grossly overweight), the Girl Scout cookies had been oddly untempting to me. I think the noneating, constant workout program puts your entire body into shock, and it just gives up completely. Anyway, I offered up the cookies. My compatriots were shocked, horrified—and, like me, completely uninterested. Starvation really does work as an appetite suppressant, it turns out.

On the last day, just before you leave, everyone gets weighed, to see how much you lost. On the "extra food" diet, I'd lost seven pounds in one week. (Compare this with the time I went

Eternally Hot

People who do yoga all the time, in general, have fantastic bodies, and they don't look their age. As compared with, say, aging gym-goers or aging runners, who have fantastic bodies but do look more their age, on average. Just an observation from an admittedly biased source.

French Women Don't Talk About Being (or Feeling) Fat

I think the key to feeling sexy and attractive is simply never voicing your doubts. If you don't say it, you won't feel it. Were I to diet, I would keep it completely secret. There's no situation that the words *I feel so fat* will improve in any way.

I also have a theory that there's a (female) hormone that makes you feel fat, regardless of the reality. The whole bloating thing surrounding your period seems overblown; I think, instead, that some nasty hormone starts floating around in greater concentrations, and everyone—the superskinny, the huge, the middling—all get this odd, new body consciousness/awareness that convinces them they're suddenly, horrifyingly fat. A few days later, you're back to normal.

So I say keep it to yourself. Those French women sure do.

on the three-hundred-calorie-a-day Cambridge diet in college; neither I nor my co-dieter Julia cheated for two weeks; she lost nine pounds, and I lost two.) The screenwriter had lost fifteen pounds (it's not fair about men and diets); everyone was happy. Even the Hollywood wives looked relieved, if only for a moment. Only the loud, self-obsessed woman with the perfect body to begin with was unhappy. She weighed 127, and she explained that her husband felt she looked good only at 126. "At 125 I'm too skinny, and at 127 I'm too fat!" she wailed (I mean, she was actually crying and close to hysterical). The rest of us exchanged ever so slightly satisfied glances: Anyone that annoying deserves a husband like that.

For all that it was pure, unmitigated torture, the Ashram

The Least You Can Do and Get Away with It

Shortly after we each had children, my friend Jennifer and I decided an in-depth, investigative piece needed to be written for *Elle* on what we felt was suddenly the most important beauty/fitness issue we could think of: How little exercise can you do and still have a decent body? Most exercise gurus, like most nutritionists, have plenty of ideas on how you could become technically perfect, if you just worked hard enough—that is, devoted your life to it, used an actual half-cup measure to portion out your daily allowance of whole-grain pasta, made sure your serving of wild salmon approximated the size of a deck of cards, never went to Krispy Kreme, drank eight glasses of water, walked, strength-trained, pushed, pulled, cross-trained, and in general simply lived at the gym. (P.S.: Why do all those advice givers have either [1] enormous thighs, [2] strained, wizened faces, or [3] a combination of the two?) You needing to improve certainly helps keep them in business.

They didn't want to answer our questions at all at first, but we grilled them and grilled them and got them all to admit (they did seem to agree, when pressed) that if you work out in some comprehensive way (some weight lifting, some moving-around sort of activity) twice a week, you can maintain your current shape and perhaps even improve on it a bit. We were not looking for weight loss, we were not looking to fit into a bikini in just ten days, we were not looking to cure heart disease or cancer. Twice a week, and you're not backsliding, and over time things can even get better. So there.

was by far the most useful and lasting, life-lesson-wise. Whenever I'm on a run or in a yoga class and I feel I can't go on, I think of standing in the boiling midday sun at the bottom of some towering ridge we were supposed to climb up, weak, starving, constipated, and cranky, and how somehow it turned out that I did have it in me and I did make it to the top, despite everything. Similarly, there was a night that they tired of lecturing us about the benefits of ingesting no food, ever, and instead had the screenwriter attempt to lift a series of weights. When we scoffed at him and said things like "No way, you can't do it, it's too heavy," despite the fact that he knew and understood we were only mouthing what they'd told us to say, he couldn't lift the weight. And when we were instructed instead to yell encouragement and praise, every time, no matter how heavy the weight, he could lift it. It wasn't exactly EST, but it worked for me, epiphany-wise.

The final spa, Green Valley in southern Utah, was lovely—the mountains there are particularly gorgeous, all rugged red and Grand Canyon–like—but I was too advanced by that point. I could hike even the instructors under the table, and I did, because I couldn't stand to hear another person detail their issues about food, which is all anyone talks about at a spa, even the instructors. I did make two important discoveries, however.

On the spa menu (various workouts, all sorts of massages, etc.), you had the choice of seeing a nutritionist. I've always suspected that nutritionists, like mean nail-salon ladies, will always tell you that you need nutritional reform no matter what shape you're actually in. Further, I think they have a devastatingly simple m.o., one that would be easy to do yourself in the privacy of your own home, for free: They query you on what your favorite foods might be, then snap back at you with a diet plan that forbids precisely those foods. Perhaps this sweeping generalization leaves out some genuinely thoughtful, knowledgeable nutritionists; I have not met them, nor have I read their commentary in magazines. You know what they're going to say before you read it: Should I eat the cheeseburger at the barbeque? Or might some crunchy celery sticks with peanut butter be a better choice?

In any case, I decided to test out my rogue theories: As I say, my body was perfect after weeks on end of starving and exercising at spas.

The nutritionist did have to work hard. I was in good shape, and the diet I claimed to adhere to (lies and more lies) was also perfect and healthy in every way. After even a cursory reading of a single *Self* magazine, anyone knows to say they eat a lot of leafy green vegetables and plenty of whole grains and not much else. So that's what I said, throwing in the occasional burrito as my supposed "occasional splurge" item. The nutritionist, after writing down all my wild claims, and noting my various weights and measurements, was perplexed; he stared at his forms long and hard. Finally he spoke. He felt I needed to work on converting some of my white fat to brown fat, which would involve various complex and nitpicky dietary changes, plus more exercise. I needed to eat fewer burritos. "I mean, on the whole, you're in great shape, I'd just like you to . . ." So the next time the nutritionist tells you you're a mess, remember, they're not going to get any money if you're in perfect health.

The other thing was the relaxation room. All spas should have a relaxation room like the one at Green Valley. It's full of plants and comfy sofas and every lame self-help book and heavily pictorial decorating book ever written. You're supposed to lounge in it while you're waiting for your treatment, but everyone just suited up in the fluffy white robes and sat in there all day. It was heaven. The faint classical music played, the estrogen flowed, the lemon and lime slices floated in the giant communal water dispenser like sleepy bathers in a warm, rippleless sea.

Relax, Honey!

Stress may indeed be the root of all human suffering; it is certainly the root of a million sorry-ass marketing ideas. The idea that your bathtub or shower can transform into a spa is as old as the original Calgon formula. It's not a bad idea; it's not even entirely untrue. My bathtub/shower was never a spa until I had children, and the second I did, it became the only place on earth where I could be alone and no one could touch me or need me or even strike up a conversation. The bath gels and the scrubs and the particular scent of a given shampoo all now send me into the Zen-ish, "not there" sort of ecstasy that I'm always trying for—but never achieving—in yoga class.

Relaxation that you've planned on is a wonderful thing; forced relaxation is one of the more stressful things there is, and it is the fate of the beauty editor. What is a spa service? A *luxury.* Who has the money to pay for luxuries? People *in a hurry.* The zeal with which day spas have embraced the New Age (perhaps better termed the Middle Age) is both comic and tragic. The same attendants who purse their lips and shake their heads over the state of one's skin, hair, or nails now dispense a similar sort of scorn over the state of one's spirit.

Being in a hurry is one of the most damnable offenses: One might as well swig whiskey while attempting to charm a member of the clergy. You arrive at a salon for a pedicure, and you know you've got a certain amount of time and a great amount of that time is going to have to be devoted to polish drying before reinserting your foot into your shoe. And they start in with the "Relax!" and the reflexology and the flower petals. "Oh, I didn't know I was getting reflexology," you say, and they smile and say, "Oh, relax, honey." If you want to charge me for something relaxing, invent some kind of New Age–y ritual for while the polish is drying, huh?

Day Spas

The greatest day spa on earth is Ten Thousand Waves in Santa Fe, New Mexico. The treatments are wonderful, but not the reason to go there: You climb up a thousand winding steps in the New Mexican dust with the piñons and the tumbleweeds all around, each step lit with a little Japanese lantern, and you wind your way up and you go to the private hot tub you've reserved for, like, $40 or something, and you sit in that hot tub with whichever operative you've chosen, and you watch the sun set from a vantage point not unlike the glorious one at the Santa Fe Opera, and the sunset is every color you've ever imagined and so wildly dramatic that it would seem to be fiction, and then you watch the moon rise over the snow-covered piñons and you get too hot in the water and you lie out on the Japanese wooden deck and you get back in—and any treatment that follows is icing on a cake that just doesn't get better, anywhere. And you write run-on sentences and there's nothing for it.

I felt that after such a soak in a Ten Thousand Waves hot tub, my husband, Gary, might feel more comfortable getting a massage—a treatment he had always feared. "What if something . . . *happens*?" he used to say.

"Like what?"

"Like, like, you know, *something*?" He would nod in the direction of his belt buckle.

I arranged for us to get a couples massage—you're both in the same room, each getting your massage from a different person. After the hot tub, they took us to this airy, cedar-cabin-fresh-air kind of room, and the wind wafted through, and I was practically falling asleep, it felt so good, when suddenly I heard giggling. And more nervous, edgy giggling. And finally, "Could you not . . . massage . . . that particular spot?" He's never had a massage since.

In their reflexive way of stating the obvious ("Feeling sick? See your doctor!"), magazine articles always tell you to look for clean, professional spa facilities. I have to speak out, however, in favor of the seedier, lower-rent spa. Though I can get free treatments at the fanciest spas in the city, I spend $80 to go to a grimy Korean day spa in a strip mall in New Jersey. For the $80, you get a sauna, a steambath, meditation, an intense full-body scrub and massage, and a facial; they even wash your hair for you. Most of all, they leave you alone; they're impersonal. The way the Turkish bath ladies ignored our screams and wild laughter. They don't care if you're relaxed or not, which for me is the most relaxing thing of all. For a little grime, they really couldn't care less about you, which in the end is all I want. Enough with the rose petals—but that's me.

The only exception to this rule is nail salons, where the cheaper you go, the more judgmental and critical the nail lady will be of your nails. If other languages are involved, she will hoot and sneer loudly with her co-workers while gesturing at you in exasperation. I am willing to pay a lot to avoid this situation.

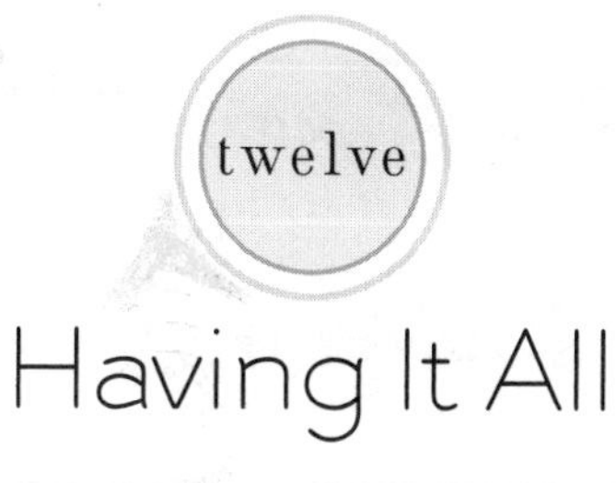

Having It All

You read about them in magazines: the women who've got a great job and a husband and gorgeous kids. There's a theme here, and by this point it may be a little alarming, but if a given lifestyle is depicted favorably in magazines, it's a good bet that I'll try to shoehorn myself into it. The J. Geils song "My Angel Is the Centerfold" always puzzled me, since, were I the narrator, finding my onetime girlfriend "on the cover of a magazine" would make my blood run hot, not cold.

I did not want to get married, particularly—perhaps because, at age twenty, I was still reading *Mademoiselle*, which sang the praises of being single. But I acquiesced—there's always divorce, I reasoned, child of 1970s Northern California that I was—and got very lucky.

Which I've come to believe is the secret of marriage: It's a crapshoot. You can live with someone for years, you can rush in after two dates—you'll never really know until after you're actually married.

Children are a much deeper commitment. If, childless, a couple decides to divorce, there's a chance they'll never have to see each other again. Having a child together—if you have any sort of humanity at all—means you're going to be in each other's lives forever, no matter how acrimonious the terms of your split-up.

For ten years, my poor husband tried everything to convince me to have a baby. There was a stuffed monkey he bought at a ski lodge; every so often I'd walk into the living room to find him on the sofa with his arm around the monkey, pretending to watch television with it. "Look! There's Mom!" he'd say, pointing at me. Unsurprisingly, I'd flee.

I liked working past 10:00 p.m. I liked movies and restaurants and bars and the sense that you get, walking aimlessly through New York, that anything is possible, that something new and surprising is just around the corner.

On our tenth anniversary, in much the resigned spirit with which I'd agreed to get married, I agreed to have a baby. Murphy's law being what it is, I got pregnant immediately.

I expected pregnancy to be one long, fat slog of ugliness and shattered dignity. That's what they tell you in the magazines, no? Strangely, it was not. The weight gain part of pregnancy turns out to be, like marriage, a crapshoot. I normally eat an enormous amount of food and, like everyone else, could stand to lose five or ten pounds. I ate truly incredible amounts of food when I was pregnant, and I gained barely twenty pounds. People I know who ate hardly a thing gained fifty. The takeaway here, I think, is that since your body is on some weird sort of autopilot and it's going to gain exactly as much as it wants to, you can actually relax about it for the first time in your life. What can you do? You're not going to make the cover of the *Sports Illustrated* swimsuit issue this year no matter what happens.

I also got the glow that everyone talks about (there's more blood flowing through your system, so your capillaries are fuller, even the ones close to the surface, so your skin glows), my hair was thicker, and all traces of acne disappeared from my face. Bobbi Brown theorizes that your lips get puffier as well.

Somewhere I read that women look good pregnant because of evolution—that if you looked hot enough, your caveman husband wouldn't desert you and would stick around to provide for you, and the baby'd be more likely to survive.

I like this theory so much better than the old familiar, she had those kids, and wow, did she go to pot.

The morning sickness was a liability on the job, unfortunately. Morning sickness occurs most often in the first few months, before you've told anyone. Scent of any sort is repulsive. One morning, I got in a cab to go to a Versace breakfast. It careened uptown, swerving wildly. The breakfast was for a new perfume, and they'd impregnated the velvet pillows we sat on with the new, heady, floral-Oriental scent. I looked down, but there was a plate of slick, steaming scrambled eggs. I looked up, and the wildly Versace'd PR person was spritzing at me.

Things got worse when I stepped into the second cab of the day to go downtown to Aveda. This cabdriver was of the lurch school of driving: Accelerate forcefully, then slam on the breaks. Repeat. I could barely stand by the time I made it to Aveda. Once inside, I found that they were promoting a new, custom, make-your-own-scent service. They divided the assembled beauty editors into small groups and rotated the groups around to a series of stations, each with many little bottles, all of them filled with separate, different fragrances to be smelled, considered carefully, and then mixed, before your eyes, into your personal combination.

Halfway through the first station, I had to sit down. The new-car smell of the cab, the Versace velvet pillows, the Versace scrambled eggs, and the nine thousand Aveda options were all swirling in my stomach. "I think I'm coming down with the flu," I lied. "Could you just describe the scents to me instead of me trying all of them?"

They began running down the list of scents and ingredients, but even thinking about all the smells made me feel woozy. I sat back down.

"I love the way Aveda shampoo smells," I finally said to the frustrated perfume mixer, who by that time was simply listing classes of ingredients to see if I liked *anything*: "Spices? Flowers? Fruits?" "Could you custom-make me a perfume that smells exactly like it?" By Aveda shampoo, I meant their best-selling Shampure; he did make a scent out of it, and to this day I've gotten more compliments on it than on any other perfume.

Men still look at you when you're pregnant, but it's a much more enjoyable experience because you know they're ogling you not in that "hey, piece of ass, I'm a man, you second-class citizen, you" sort of way, but in that appreciative, "I love women" way you encounter in Italy. Instead of the usual implied assault, the look seems to telegraph a modicum of respect.

If you happen to luck out and look good while you're pregnant, everyone will tell you you're having a boy. People would stop me in the street to inform me I was having a boy. I of course had a girl, then, the second time around, a boy. A girl steals your beauty, is the old wives' tale. Not to turn this book into a feminist tract, but come on.

My new, extreme vanity got me into trouble, naturally. Long before I was pregnant, I had a pair of Prada loafers that were simply gorgeous. They were just plain black loafers, but there was *something* about them; men, women, and children would stare at them in the street. Everyone asked me where I got them. They were fabulous, and that was that. I was standing in line at the Duane Reade one day when I was about eight months pregnant, wearing the loafers. "Those are great shoes," said the man behind me, his voice full of the genuine admiration the shoes never failed to inspire. I was reading the label on the pregnancy vitamins, so I didn't even look up.

"Thank you," I said.

"I love the leather," he continued.

"It's great, isn't it?" I was smiling, still looking at the vitamin label, overaccustomed to adulation.

"Could I see the label—on—on the inside?" he asked. I was secretly proud of the fact that the label on the inside was in fact "Prada"; I slid my foot right out to ever so modestly display the label.

The man was oddly silent. After a moment or so, I finally looked up. He was staring at the shoe and my foot, frozen the way a cat becomes paralyzed after a few swipes past a sprig of catnip. Disheveled in that clearly mentally-ill way. I dropped the vitamins on the floor and ran out of the store.

A New Life

However beautiful you feel or don't feel while pregnant, the ugliness of having been pregnant two weeks ago is truly horrifying. You're sagging and lumpy, your hair's unkempt and falling out, you've had no sleep in two weeks so your eyes look like your eighty-year-old grandmother's, your skin is ashen, and everyone's sick to death of you and your crying baby.

I wore hideous plaid pajamas, my hair fell into the same tangled mat that hadn't been seen since seventh grade, I developed rashy scabs all over my neck. Like the plainswoman in the

Baby Presents

If your friend's had a baby, don't buy millions of presents or even make special gourmet dinners. Come over and hold the baby so she can sleep. Or send her for a massage or a facial, again while you hold the baby. Or hold the baby and address all the envelopes for her thank-you notes. Tell her she looks incredibly hot and let her sleep.

Dorothea Lange portrait, without the dignity. I mumbled and shuffled around the apartment, listless yet angry, deeply unappealing. I guess the evolution thing applies only until the baby is technically outside of your body—then the baby starts working its own, much more adorable survival-of-the-fittest charms on everyone, and you become somewhat extraneous.

The thing, I found out, is not to consider your appearance for six weeks. They say nine months in, nine months out, but after six weeks much of your prepregnant self returns, particularly if you breast-feed. Breast-feeding, besides being fantastic for the baby and preventing breast cancer for you, is like working out on a treadmill six or eight or however many times you do it a day. It leaves you incredibly skinny, with enormous breasts.

After six weeks is when the doctors say you can have sex again (not that it was appealing to me at that point in any way), so maybe there is something to my whole evolution-pregnancy-non-pregnancy attractiveness idea. If, in theory, you might technically be able to reproduce, the gods will shine their lights back down upon you.

Going back to work is hard, but being a full-time stay-at-home mom is much harder. This statement naturally reflects *my* feelings about *my* work situation, and I doubt I'd have written the same sentence if I worked, say, in a vinyl flooring factory in southern New Jersey, took the bus home every night, and then set back out for my second job waitressing at the diner. But for the privileged women for whom work is a choice, I stand by my words. Work provides you with all sorts of positive (and negative) reinforcement—Good job! We hated it! We loved it! Approved! whatever—plus an alternate identity, an artifact of the old you, to cling to. You get dressed up and put on a little M•A•C and go to work, and it's like a genius disguise that fools everyone. You come home, and your child is thrilled to see you, and you're thrilled to see your child. I know it's different for everyone, but there it is.

It's a weird balancing act (curse *Redbook* for ever running that "Juggler" ad campaign that makes anyone cringe when discussing this subject), but for me there was something fun about trying to do everything. Maybe rats on treadmills are enjoying themselves, after all.

Does Walking Actually Work?

It takes longer, but it keeps you in just as good shape as running, and this is how I know: Normally a runner (I was not yet into yoga), I walked while I was pregnant. It took forever, but running just felt awkward and uncomfortable, even though the doctor said it was okay. Six weeks after having the baby, I ventured out for a run. I hadn't run in at least nine months. I ran four miles, no problem.

It was harder to keep up with the fabulousness, however. The nights with the mandatory black-tie events, for instance. While I'd still borrow something good from the fashion closet, the free makeup job and hairstyling appointments all went by the wayside. I'd rush home from work, play play play, make-dinner-put-to-bed-chat-with-sitter-put-on-borrowed-clothes-slap-on-lipstick-hop-in-a-cab-at-the-last-minute, and then I'd realize on the way there that not only was my hair not done, but there was spit-up in it. "Oh, you smell so good," some black-tie operative would invariably comment. I'd arrive back home just as India was stirring and starting to scream in terror at the sight of the last-minute sitter but instead saw me and went back to sleep. It was exhausting, but I liked it.

It was not quite enough, though; I needed more time with her. They're only the age they are once, was my feeling. So when we moved out of the city and into crunchy suburbia, I threatened to quit and thus successfully negotiated a four-day work week.

I know, when I look around, how lucky I am in having been able to make this arrangement work. But no one talks about working mothers who *don't* have it bad: It's like bragging about how much money you make, or how great you are. I think that's one of the reasons it's so rare. All the articles focus on the mom who can barely pay for day care now that they've slashed her salary and benefits, or the mom who never sees her kids because she leaves before dawn and gets home at midnight and makes millions but loses out on life. But explaining how you work three days a week (I know several women who do precisely this, P.S.) *and* make good money is just unseemly, somehow on a par with the WorldCom scandal, smacking of entitlement, so no one talks about it. If they did talk about it, perhaps it would become more common, and the world might become a better place.

My advice re: that is to wait until you've had the baby, so you know precisely what you want and what you're willing to give up if you don't get it. And when you're negotiating the fewer days thing, ask yourself, Are you going to be doing any less work? So should they pay you less money? In my case, the beauty section in the magazine was certainly not getting any smaller; I was not going to be writing, editing, or going to events any less; nor were they hiring additional people to pick up the slack.

Crunchy Suburbia

I chose my particular suburb for its unsuburbanness: its artists, organic food co-ops, diversity, etc. And while I wouldn't trade it for a Junior League/crewneck sweater/blond highlights kind of suburb, it has its peccadillos.

Nyack, New York, sits across the Hudson River from Westchester County—the well-manicured, keeping-up-with-the-Joneses site of John Cheever intrigue. Nyack is the bohemian, hippie/alterna/ultra-PC option. The bad bumper stickers (THE ONLY GOOD BUSH IS MY OWN) proliferate like fruit flies; the pressure to appear nonconformist is intense and unrelenting.

Once, after a few drinks at the now defunct Coven Café (when I saw *Blair Witch,* I was even more horrified than I might have been, because I recognized all the weird markings and dangly things from my hikes in the woods all around Nyack, which turns out to be the Wiccan capital of America), I looked around at all the Judy Chicago posters and offered my friend Lisa $100 if she would wear a pair of Chanel sunglasses (beauty giveaway, natch) in town for an entire day. She declined.

To do so would have completely destroyed her image: "I was really disappointed today, honey."

"Oh why, sweetheart?"

"Well, I saw Lisa D. at the farmer's market in these—awful . . . designer sunglasses—big flashy logos all over them, just awful. I just never thought she was that kind of person." Some Nyack person would have actually said this; I'd stake my life on it.

My image is already shot—I work for a magazine whose sole purpose is to encourage people to buy more things—and still, I won't wear the sunglasses, either. Adam and his (black) boyfriend were mobbed, celebrity style, when they took the kids to the park one day: Black! Gay! If only one of them had been formerly incarcerated, or perhaps lactose intolerant, they could have really ruled. And perhaps I, by association, might've moved up in the standings.

The crunchy suburbia look affects utter freedom from vanity. No makeup, no obvious blow-dries, lots of peasant skirts and interesting beadwork. Ponchos are big, mascara is not. A woman needs a man like a fish needs a bicycle.

Early on, Lisa and I decided to throw a party together; we had it at my house. The only problem was the hulking large-screen TV in my living room (it was so large that the previous owners had been unable to figure out a way to get it out of the house to take it with them). As we sat waiting for our guests to arrive, we took bets on how many people we'd catch whispering to one another in horror at the TV. I won: six separate whispering-in-horror incidents in the course of one three-hour party. "Um, did you see . . . you know, uh, *that*?"

"My God, did you see . . . *the* . . . ?"

We had the party at her house the next year.

I grew up in crunchy suburbia; before Palo Alto, California, became the red hot nexus of all Internet profiteering and greed (and the hottest real estate market in the country), it was a hotbed of boycotts and pro-Che bumper stickers. I know and fully recognize the power of a beat-up ten-year-old Volvo.

So I feel at home in my town, though I find myself shunned or at least frowned upon by many of the townspeople. There's the Brobdingnagian TV that looms over my living room. There's my vanity-centric day job and my car—though it is used and many years old, a BMW is a BMW is a yuppie statusmobile any way you slice it.

I flip back and forth every day: drop my daughter off at school, my hair unbrushed, face bare, jeans rent, shirt full of holes; race back for a *Mommie Dearest* makeup-and-hair moment while my son plays with lotion samples on the floor; make the perfume-launch doughnuts all day, flouncing around in car-service cars and Manolo Blahniks; arrive home and get back into the jeans, tone down the makeup, mess up my hair, and go out to the Women's Creative Collective Craft Bazaar and live it up.

"You purposely make yourself ugly!" admonishes Adam. "Would it kill you to try to look pretty? Why do you care what the Villagers think?"

For all their holistic modesty, the Villagers are a randy bunch; perhaps it is always this way in suburbs, I don't know. There are three-ways here and wild affairs there. People are constantly discovering new facets of their sexuality. And of course everyone else finds out, so it's very high school.

Though I loathe facials, I was thrilled to be invited to a facial party at the local midwife's house (P.S.: The midwife later delivered my son); there were bagels and tea and an enormous chocolate cake, and people seemed to have forgotten the TV and overlooked the BMW enough that I'd made the cut. A woman named Heidi was doing the facials, which involved washcloths steeped in a vast communal pot (this did give me pause; the water was brown, murky, and speckled with random herbs in a way that both looked and smelled like a limpid broth of, say, turnips) and applications of various salves and oils (like anyone prone to breakouts, I'm mortally afraid of any sort of oil being worked into my face), while we all sat around a big table, our hair tied back with scarves, gossiping about everyone else in town.

One woman was talking about how hard her stay-at-home-dad husband was "working" for a local antiques dealer (everyone except her correctly suspected they were having a wild affair). Another woman jokingly went on about how hot the organic farmgirls at the farmer's market were (she was already sleeping with one of them). It was a good thing we all had washcloths over our faces.

As I sat there, relaxed and happy despite the drama and the oils and the communal pot, I realized why I've always hated facials: (1) You're alone in some antiseptic room. (I think the alone part is the worst for me; I lie there blindfolded by some eye mask, thinking to myself that I don't know the aesthetician at all and how easy it'd be, were they to have Jeffrey Dahmer–like tendencies, to simply slit my throat; but that's another story.) (2) The aesthetician's (murderous or not) attention is focused entirely on you and the dire state of your skin. (3) The only escape from the scathing criticisms of the aesthetician is to buy six zillion dollars' worth of product right then and there.

Fending Off the Facial Lady

The truth is, you can't. The only truly effective strategy is to pretend not to speak English, and even then you'll probably get an elaborate pantomime about the proper skin care and where you might buy it (from her, of course). Magazines always advise simply stating that you want to relax, so you'd rather not talk. In my experience, it takes bigger guns than that. Something along the lines of, "My boyfriend and I just broke up, and if you say anything, I'm going to cry." Or the thing I wish I had the balls to do: Take out a $20 bill (or whatever's an appropriate but on the high side tip) and say, "Here's your tip. Every time you say something to me, I'm taking away five dollars."

We all bought something from Heidi (the facial lady), but it was so much more pleasant with the cake and the gossip and the freedom from judgment—at least judgment over the state of our skin.

Eventually, I developed a gang of not-quite-crunchy-or-suburban-enough friends (one husband refers to us as "the Witches of Nyack"). Together, we've come up with a variety of strategies for coping with the PC-ness and the high school–ness of it all. The Witches went through a big gymnastics phase; ostensibly, we drove all the way into the city because we wanted to be in better shape, but the real reasons were more interesting. If yoga is all about peace, and aerobics is all about the burn, the vibe you get at an adult gymnastics class is one of pure, wanton sexuality. You might not expect such a thing—the term *adult gymnastics class* sounds dopily clunky and remedial—but there it is.

I am no gymnast, adult or otherwise; dopily clunky and remedial is closer to the truth. My girlfriends, on the other hand, flip and tuck and roll and whirl like a pack of twelve-year-old dervishes on the Romanian Olympic team. And when they started driving in to the Chelsea Piers gym twice a week, it was flip and tuck or sacrifice what small social life I'd managed to carve out for myself. "You'll be fine!" they insisted. "It's easy!"

Needless to say, they started in with double-back-handspring backflip layouts, and I was left to practice my only skill, the cartwheel, over and over again—adrift in the roiling sea of chalk dust and sexual tension, hot guys flipping in one direction and hot girls flying by in another.

If you're not quite sure you can pull off the triple somersault whatever, you get a spot from one of the finely muscled, much-lusted-over instructors. The cutest ones always had a line of eager students waiting for a spot. The fellow students (some of them equally hot) were wildly encouraging, clapping and shrieking for even the most faintly successful attempt at a handstand. All in all, the whole overheated atmosphere added up to a huge ego boost for everyone involved.

Buoyed by all the flirting, praise, and general cuteness (not to mention the many spots), I managed to do several back handsprings, thrillingly but foolishly.

Perhaps equally foolish, we followed up every workout with a trip across the West Side Highway to one of several bars, where we knocked back mojitos with the cute instructors and fellow students. One of the Witches is a famous actress, which we tend to forget until we're out in some bar and people start coming up for autographs, adding to the surreal quality of the atmosphere and introducing us to more operatives than we might otherwise meet (it takes some alcohol to get your average Manhattanite to come up and ask someone for an autograph, so most of the people we met were preselected for bad behavior). Things progressed: We went from bars to dance clubs; we stayed out later, alarming the husbands. It's the worst sort of cliché, a group of fortyish suburban gals pretending to be New York City club kids, knocking back shots, and throwing themselves at perplexed gymnastics instructors. But we did have fun.

The calories we burned in the gymnastics we put back in with the mojitos; overall, we may have ended up looking worse, what with all the undereye bags. I think that's what keeps your average suburban mom from going completely AWOL after a few drinks—the fact that her kids are going to get her up at 6:00 a.m. no matter how late she stayed out the night before.

Getting your kicks in town has proved to be a little more work. Social activities revolve around the Nyack Center, an old church where they have the creative-women's-collective-type activities, concerts, alterna-movies, and, of course, the yearly Sweetheart Dance. The Sweetheart Dance occurs close to Valentine's Day. Crepe paper hearts strung from long skeins of red yarn trail from the rafters. People in flannel shirts and running shoes bend and twist earnestly to Van Morrison. (I cannot lose myself in dance, try as I might; my self-consciousness doubtlessly telegraphs hopeless vanity and vast insecurity, but still I can't.) The first year, we went all out, my friend Lisa and I: Instead of the expected spinach dip or chocolate-chip cookies, we decided to blow everyone away with a supercreative Indian recipe involving lentils, unusual spices, and thousands of hollowed-out mini potatoes. Healthful, multicultural . . . we

"Natural" Makeup

Cosmetics executives (male ones) are forever admonishing all the beauty editors: "Why don't you wear makeup?!!" To me, this is a variant on my least favorite male street comment: "Smile, honey!" It also shows how clueless they are about how their customers operate and what their customers, at the end of the day, might want.

I think I may be the winner in the "no makeup" makeup category, simply because of the Nyack factor, where an errant glob of mascara might trigger the question "Are you *wearing makeup*?!" (delivered in the tone one might use to say, "Are you *molesting children*?!") that could send you to social Siberia—or at least Westchester—for the rest of your days.

Anyway, the ingredients:

1. Mascara, one coat. Use your fingers to disperse any clumps, or if you're particularly fastidious, use a Q-tip dipped in makeup remover. Either way, do the mascara first, so it doesn't smudge up anything else you've put on.

2. Tinted moisturizer. Think sheer, sheer, sheer. Your freckles should show. If you're oily, use blotting sheets.

3. Spend the majority of your time applying concealer—red and brown spots, undereye circles—and blending it carefully, carefully, carefully. I'll repeat: Pat, don't rub. That phrase was almost the title of this book.

4. You might want a little eye cream on the outer corners of your eyes—it sort of softens everything.

5. Clear, not-too-shiny lip balm.

made about six hundred of them, and I think maybe about three were eaten.

We applied our makeup carefully, so it would appear that we weren't wearing a thing; we didn't touch our hair, so as to maintain the "I've slept on this for three days" look. Clothing for these sorts of events is all about a skirt with a pant, ideally with some sort of Central American accessory thrown in. Lisa can really work this look; it couldn't be worse on me, but I made it happen, rather than risk being stoned in the parking lot.

We stood by our potatoes, willing them to catch on and gulping beer to soothe our righteous, injured psyches, watching the Villagers get down and chow on un-PC brownies (who could blame them?). No one seemed to notice us or our gorgeous no-makeup, as long as we stood expectantly by the trays of potatoes. In the end, brownies and pigs-in-a-blanket win with everyone, even the most righteous left-wingers.

Unsurprisingly, everyone's got an acupuncturist, a massage therapist, a shaman, and a homeopath. Two of the Witches of Nyack, one of them a girl who won't go to a doctor to save her life, went through a colonic phase. Like all other colonic enthusiasts (the beauty business is full of them; makeup artists are particularly susceptible), they quickly became obsessive and prone to giving out far too much information when relating their irrigation/cleansing experiences to others. When the no-doctors friend developed a 104-degree fever one night, did she call the doctor? No, she called the colonic lady, who sagely advised her that it was simply her body ridding itself of toxins. "You'll be fine," she assured her. "Go to bed." She ended up in the hospital for close to a week.

Another Witch of Nyack prefers shamans, real ones who come up from various South American countries to visit their many Nyack fans. One night, she came back furious from an important shaman meeting: "The interpreter woman was just so nasty—she kept cutting off my access and refusing to tell me what he was saying or letting him answer my questions." She paused, fuming. "I think that woman is fucking the shaman."

A few days later, my baby-sitter mentioned that my daughter's swimming teacher wouldn't be coming that week. "She's got some . . . shaman? . . . staying at her house?" The swimming teacher was the shaman fucker! Things really come together quickly in a small town.

I make fun of it all, but where did I end up when my three-month-old son had the most awful case of eczema all over his entire body and the doctors could do nothing—other than coat him with steroids, which are no good for most people, let alone a baby? The homeopath. And how long did it take the homeopath to completely cure him of the eczema (it's never returned)? One month. Was it the homeopathic cure? "Take him off the homeopathy for a few days," she advised when I called her to report that the eczema had completely disappeared. It came back the next day. "Put him back on for another week," she said. I did, and when I stopped for the second time, it really and truly was gone forever.

The unassuming shaman-fucker has also taken note, like the many hopeful *Elle* fashion girls before her, of the handsome Adam, who is often lurking in the background during the swimming lessons—he's out at my house a great deal, especially in the summer, as he's given up on being an art director entirely and become a photographer. She's asked him out several times.

The supposedly open-minded Villagers are skeptical about the Adam arrangement. Even in these enlightened times, it seems, a man and a woman cannot be platonic friends—even if one is gay and the other married. If I had a dollar for all the raised, Al-Franken-faithful eyebrows . . .

No one could be happier about Adam being around than my children, who adore him. He's singlehandedly gotten India to look people in the eye and say "please" and "thank you" by offering to help her build Bionicals, weird plastic Lego-like monsters made for children but impossible for children to put together. He can sing endless rounds of the *Music Together* classic "Hello, Everybody" with my son, Wiley, on the floor without becoming unglued.

When he actually went to the *Music Together* class—curious after hearing all the songs ad nauseam—he found himself surrounded by eager, at times even predatory moms, shimmying before him with reckless abandon. He loves to take Wiley to the park, and he always comes home with his pockets stuffed full of phone numbers. "A three-year-old is just a woman magnet!" he exclaims. "It's just that Wiley's so cute, all those moms can't resist him." Beyond the swimming teacher, the yoga lady out-and-out asked him on a date; the moms picking up their kids from a playdate linger into the evening; certain dads are also visibly intrigued.

There's a lone gay bar in all of Rockland County—someone installed neon lights and a dance floor in an otherwise unassuming ranch house along route 9W—and Adam caused quite a stir there, too. Several indignant regulars thought his arriving in a car stuffed with child paraphernalia was a little over the top. "What's your poor wife up to while you're out carousing around?" demanded one. "Don't think we don't see the car seats in the back of that Volvo!"

We were walking back from the hardware store with the

kids one afternoon; the alarming-pro-Bush hardware store owner had given them small American flags, which they both waved enthusiastically. Adam, laden with painting supplies (horrified at the unstylish state of my house, he refinishes anything he can get his hands on), had Wiley on his shoulders and India on his arm, the flags going gangbusters, when he saw a man he once knew (doubtlessly in the biblical sense of the word) from New York. *Oh, so that's how it is now,* the man's scornful look seemed to say.

Having Adam around increased the incidences of at-home beauty moments; he is much more willing than I to believe the claims inscribed on the back of the boxes of eye creams, face serums, etc., and he is much more excited to sample things than my product-weary husband. We tried a $2,100, twenty-one-day face treatment system; then we tried an anti-dark-circle gel that promised results in two weeks. Both times, I came away vaguely pleased, hoping against hope that perhaps I was actually seeing some small effects—and he was ecstatic. This may be because he miraculously has no wrinkles to begin with; I once had to buy cigarettes for him because the deli owner was sure he was underage; at the time, I think he was about thirty-eight. He steals my self-tanner spray (Wiley greatly enjoys spraying him with it) and my acne treatments and my Retin-A. The Villagers were quietly horrified when we all (India, Wiley, Adam, and I) gave ourselves pedicures with a new dark purple polish called Drifter.

We even got Gary in on the beautifying one night when I brought home a new microdermabrasion system. The three of us sat around the table after the kids were in bed and put the peel stuff all over our faces ("It's stinging! I think it's working!") and alphahydroxy cream all over our feet. Gary went along with it, attempting (in vain) to teach us how to play poker while we waited.

Adam shares in my amazement over India's militant anti-glamour sensibilities: Ever since she was a baby, she was loathe to so much as touch a doll; she'd visibly recoil if presented with one. Wrangling her into a dress usually requires both bribes and force.

She's also clearly drunk from the Village water, as Adam found out when he took her to the Plaza for lunch one day when she was about six. "Let's have a cocktail, why don't we?" he began.

"Adam," she said, in her all-business way. "I am a child. I cannot drink alcoholic beverages."

"No, what I mean is, let's have a Shirley Temple."

"Who is Shirley Temple?" (I'm very anti-TV. I just am. I think two-year-olds who can perform entire Britney Spears routines are sad, not cute. I loathe irony in a child; children have not yet had the experiences that might entitle them to the jadedness that most kids' shows I've seen encourage. I know anti-TV-ers send pro-TV-ers over the edge in exasperation, but there it is.)

After the Shirley Temple drink was brought and happily consumed, and the particulars of the actual Shirley Temple were explained (the fame, the movies, the dancing, the singing, the curls, the cuteness), India spent the rest of the day casting aspersions.

"All Shirley cares about are her ringlets and her tap shoes!"

"I bet she wore makeup even though she was a little girl!"

"All she did was run around trying to please MEN!"

"Where does she get it?" Adam wanted to know. "I know it's not you. What are they teaching at that school of hers?"

One day, my parents were cleaning out their attic and sent me the doll I had loved most as a child, the Sasha doll, a Euro-ish girl of seemingly Nordic origin, clearly from the seventies, with dark, dark skin and white-blond hair (the characteristics, as I've mentioned, that I worshipped at the time). Being a doll, Sasha was stridently ignored by India until, in the hands of Adam, Sasha became Courtley Bacon. Under his tutelage, she acquired a huffy, Aunt Jemima sort of accent and a severe manner. She is called in for serious child misbehavior: fighting, whining, going near the stove, breaking toys, that sort of thing. Her blistering lectures are feared above all else: "Now, Wiley June, you sit down in that chair and you *think* about what you just said to your sister!"

"But Courtley, I—"

"Don't you 'I Courtley' me! You sit in that chair and you *think* and you APOLOGIZE! On the double!"

○

There are alternative films and documentaries shown at the Nyack Center. One night, Gary didn't want to go, and Adam had been shooting all day, so I convinced him to come with me. That day, at work, I'd finally tried out a spray-tanning booth. Spray tans are quick, to be sure, but there's the down-time involved in actually going to the spray tan place, so it took a long time for me to finally make it happen. I locked myself into the booth, the machine sprayed (kind of gross, and it's a little disconcerting breathing the fumes), and I blended, dried, and went back to the office, promptly forgetting about it.

I was late getting home from work, so I barely had time to exchange my heels for work boots and my shimmery, *Lucky*-girl top for a sweater full of moth holes before I drove with Adam quickly to the Nyack Center to meet up with my friends.

Spray Tan Caveats

The forty-second spray tan booth is brilliant, especially if you have to be on a beach in the near future. The lengthier, forty-minute, aesthetician-administered spray tan is going to be a little better, but not so much that it's worth the extra time and expense.

- Ignore the attitude of the attendants. Why they think you need to be ashamed of yourself is beyond me.
- Put regular body lotion on your palms, your ankles, your toes (especially the cuticles), your elbows, and your nipples or you risk darkening those areas in an unflattering and disconcerting way.
- If you see a streak as you step out, blend immediately and furiously.

The documentary, the must-watch *Keep the River on Your Right,* was brilliant (on cannibalism, primitivism, aging, and the enduring greatness of New York City), and it featured the incredible, amazing music of Steven Bernstein (Nyack resident). We emerged delighted, in something of a daze, feeling at last a part of the smart alterna-crowd that now mixed in the postfilm discussion area.

But I caught a glimpse of myself in a mirror along the hallway (I know, narcissism at its most extreme) and saw, to my horror, that the forgotten spray tan had at last taken effect—and I was a perfectly toasty *Baywatch*/Playboy Channel bronze from head to toe. I radiated the sort of seamless, tanned perfection you rarely see outside of soft-porn videos and diet infomercials. Not a look for the politically correct in the dead of winter. "Adam," I said in a harsh whisper, flattening my back

Self-Tanning DIY

While there's no pill to instantly make someone look slimmer and younger, if you're at all pale, there is a lotion. Self-tanner drastically minimizes exhaustion, undereye bags, blotchy skin, and cellulite. It's possible that none of this is true and that I have some kind of body dysmorphic disorder brought on by a casual comment by my old boyfriend: "You'd be really gorgeous if you were tan . . . like Casey." Casey was the most beautiful girl ever at Stanford, worshipped by all, who took her bronzed stardom even further when she appeared naked in the campus production of *Hair*.

- In my opinion, the much-talked-about exfoliation step isn't so important. A shower and towelling-off should do it for most people.
- Tinted self-tanner makes the whole endeavor about nine hundred times easier—you can see the spots you missed.
- Spend lots of time blending.
- Your feet are the biggest challenge and probably the one area that you might want to think about really exfoliating. Beyond that, the body lotion step mentioned in "Spray Tan Caveats" is critical. If you forget, you can put the lotion on those spots immediately after the self-tanner.
- Wash your hands when you're through, then put a blob of tanner on the back of one hand and rub the backs of your hands together.
- Ignore the instructions about not getting dressed. Put on some dark-colored clothes and go about your business. Who wants to sit around in the bathroom naked, shivering, and feeling ridiculous?
- If your tan has to be perfect, do it a few days before it's going to be on display and come back in the next day to fix any mistakes.

against the wall. "We've got to go." He looked at me, of course, as if I were crazy. "Don't you want to hang out and talk to everyone?"

"Look at me!" I pointed at my face. His face was blank. "I'm tan!" He still looked confused. "Too tan!" True friend that he was, he hightailed it out of there with me, laughing loudly at my ridiculousness, but I did not care. I had escaped with my life, if not my pride.

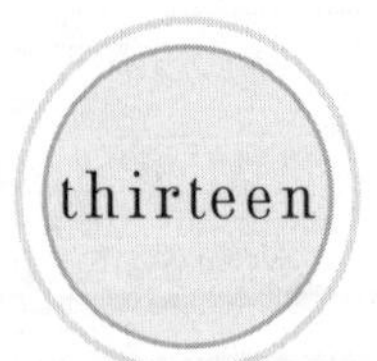

The Signs of Aging—and the Desperate Measures I Took

The carnival, one might be tempted to assume, is a thing of the past (I'm talking carny carnival—cotton candy and old sticky metal Ferris wheels, not Venice or anything involving a masked ball): something for edgy photographers to shoot fashion pictures in, a place fraught with irony and nostalgia, failed Americana.

But if you're a kid, the carnival is an entirely viable (indeed, impossibly fabulous) entity. So Lisa and I packed up our small charges, and off we went to the carnival. I was thirty-four, that age that you find yourself—to your surprise and delight—still, for the most part, ageless.

It was a sweltering day, unsurprisingly. We were hot to see some really choice carnies—missing teeth, cigar breath, copious greasy eyeliner. But carnies today all look like they work for Bennigan's: bright blue polo shirts, khaki shorts, clear skin, straight teeth. We found only one—a woman who shouted obscenities at the small children who attempted to get onto her ride without first taking off their shoes. "Jesus!" she said, taking a drag on her cigarette and rolling her eyes heavenward dramatically. But that was it.

One well-groomed, overly normal carny was guessing people's ages; he barked at us as we went past. "Hey, *MISS BLISS!"* he yelled (I was wearing a T-shirt from the Bliss spa in New York). "Two dollars if I'm right!"

Okay, I thought, if anyone should be able to fool this person, it's me: I have access to every salve and youth potion known to man, and I slather it all on with reckless abandon. "Sure," I challenged.

He squinted at me. "Well, take off your sunglasses!" he roared. A crowd was gathering. "How can I tell your age without seeing around your eyes?"

Note to self: No more carnivals, ever. I took them off.

"Oh," he said, as if it were obvious to everyone, "you're thirty-four. Not that there's anything wrong with that."

The Aging Scribe

Can I just say how depressing the documentation (magazines, reality shows, etc.) of plastic surgery is? Yes, like a car wreck,

Instant Youthifier

"I love it when I break out!" exclaimed a co-worker when I complained about my teenager-y skin. "I look so young!" Indeed, a breakout is like a giant billboard screaming NOT OLD YET! right there on your face.

it is fascinating, and no, there's nothing wrong with it, but doesn't it just kill your buzz about practically everything else on earth to read the excruciating details of someone's blepharoplasty/dermabrasion experience?

The worst thing about the magazine stories are the pitted and tattered psyches of the people who write them: When you write the story of your face lift or your liposuction, you of course have to *get* the face lift or the liposuction. Of course, you'd never have gotten plastic surgery were it not, after all, *your job:* You're not at all vain or crazy or a little ridiculous, like

Liposuction

Though I know many happy liposuctionees, I still feel it's an ill-advised measure: You get rid of fat cells in one spot, and a few years later you eat a few too many Krispy Kremes and you have to get fat somewhere, and since there are no more fat cells in the spot(s) you liposuctioned, it's anybody's guess as to where you'll suddenly find yourself pudgy: your back? your calves? your cheeks? It's got to go somewhere. Plus, there's also the thing of how much difference is it going to make in your life to have an inch or so off your thighs? Is someone going to fall in love with you who otherwise wouldn't? Once you've got that inch off, when you find it hasn't really changed things, might you end up surfing that slippery slope of, Oh, maybe I'll get this taken off, too—?

The whole thing of having to wear a girdle that oozes bodily fluids for several weeks afterward is undeniably repellent, also. That and the scary *Allure* stories about people who've died getting it.

But again, I do know very satisfied liposuction customers (I'd never have guessed any of them had had it done, either), so . . .

the rest of those poor saps sitting in the waiting room; you're *on assignment.* You're a journalist! Just doing your job.

There was (still is, somewhere, God knows what she looks like now) a terrifying writer who'd spent her early years (and several articles) as the girlfriend of a prominent hairstylist and after him began writing about plastic surgery, which she naturally would have to undergo before writing about. I got about a proposal a month from this woman: liposuction, dermabrasion, eye lifts, brow lifts, collagen . . . What was even worse was that she was perfectly attractive, even youthful. A piece of hers would turn up in a given magazine, and then another, and then the editor would finally get creeped out.

"Free" and "surgery" and "audience" just don't belong together. Think of the reality shows with the poor seventeen-year-old-twins wanting to be transformed into Brad Pitt, the downtrodden moms with their weak chins and their sagging confidence . . . Ouch.

The publicists of plastic surgeons provide the clearest cautionary tale. *Allure* once ran an article where prominent plastic surgeons were photographed next to their wives; the pictures were indeed worth a thousand words. If you must have a Svengali, keep him far away from anesthesia, knives, and your face. The plastic surgeon's publicist, however, gets it even worse. Like the investigative journalists, they too do it for the free surgery. Surgeons, perhaps rightly, see the publicist as the billboard on which to showcase their work. Add money to this already incendiary equation, and the results are rarely pretty.

You might think I'm completely against plastic surgery. I think I *am* completely against cheek and lip implants; one quick perusal of awfulplasticsurgery.com should cure just about anyone hankering for either of those. The thing is, I've seen people with some very good plastic surgery—not very many of them, but they're there, and I'm sure they're going to play upon my mind as the years continue their inexorable march forward. There's one woman in the beauty industry who was always perfectly nice looking, but when she got plastic surgery (I'm thinking in her late fifties or early sixties), she was transformed into a genuinely beautiful woman. She doesn't look just younger, she looks fantastically beautiful—suddenly graceful and forgiving in the way that exceptionally beautiful women are—and everyone including me is dying to know who did it. My friend's mom got a face lift in her early fifties, and she's now seventy and she still looks fifty. Go figure.

Botox

Like everyone when they initially hear about it, I was horrified by Botox. It is literally (not figuratively) the most toxic substance on earth, meaning that it takes less of it to kill you than anything else—arsenic, anthrax, hydrochloric acid . . . anything. My sister explained this to me after I'd first been to the office of Dr. Fredric Brandt, aka the Baron of Botox—he's said to use more Botox than any other doctor on earth—to see him inject an actual patient.

Dr. Brandt himself is an energetic, wiry person of indeterminant age: Over the years, he appears to have gotten younger. He's always in a very trim, almost *Sprockets*-like ensemble by Prada or Miu Miu, punctuated by a golden bracelet studded with what look like large blue-and-black fish eyes that I've divined (by seeing similar bracelets in an article about Madonna in *US Weekly;* this kind of detective work is what I do with my spare time, sadly) was given to him by a grateful (and fabulous-looking, I must say) Madge herself. (While he will never comment, it is widely rumored that Madonna flies Dr. Brandt to London on a regular basis.)

I was surprised when I walked into Dr. Brandt's office that day, because the "patient" didn't look old to me at all. She was maybe in her mid-thirties—maybe her early thirties, really—and wanted to get rid of her crow's-feet, and she felt her neck was too wrinkled. It just looked like a neck to me, and the crow's-feet were barely visible. Dr. Brandt said he would do one side of her face first, so I could see the difference.

It's hard to watch a person getting botulism toxin injected directly into her neck. Dr. Brandt sang bits of cheery show tunes to himself as he worked, which made the whole scene all the more disturbing.

But the results were genuinely amazing: You know how some people's mouths kind of turn down all the time, so they always look a little discouraged? It turns out your neck muscles are responsible for dragging your entire face down; one side of the woman's mouth suddenly looked a little happier, a little more upbeat. The barely perceptible crow's-feet were gone—and injecting Botox there doesn't reduce your ability to make expressions, the way the between-your-brows Botox does, so it isn't always about a frozen grimace.

To finish things off, he gave her a shot above each eyebrow, miraculously lifting it (and the skin just below it) up. Incredibly beautifying—and, I had to admit, a great deal less traumatic than a surgical brow lift. And no David Guest/Janice Dickinson/Jocelyn Wildenstein permanent hawk-eyed leer, either.

For several years, I recommended Dr. Brandt to people who asked me about Botox, but I was always secretly horrified at their willingness to risk death and injury for the sake of beauty. Then one day, I, toxin-obsessed, organic-food fanatic that I am, woke up, looked in the mirror, and called that Dr. Brandt right up.

I took along Adam, who wanted to try collagen—he was hoping for "the Heather Locklear effect" under his eyes: The skin at Heather Locklear's cheekbones continues, uninterrupted, to her lower lashes with no changes in tone or texture whatsoever. (Collagen, as it turns out, is not the secret to the Heather Locklear effect—nor is anything else I've discovered, sad to say—beyond, of course, the superior genetics of Heather Locklear.)

I was going to try Botox. I made Adam go first, with the collagen. Dr. Brandt moved in breezily with his syringe, hum-

I Know, I Know

People accuse me of Howard Hughes–esque tendencies around the sun (ideally I sit under an umbrella, clothed, slick with sunscreen), but I watched my stepfather die of melanoma. Worse than death, for many people, however, are wrinkles, sagging, age spots, broken capillaries, and all the rest of it. Compare the skin on your butt with the skin on the back of your hand. Does the sun make a difference?

They recently debunked the whole "90 percent of your sun damage occurs before you're eighteen years old" myth (a myth I thought was a fact but is, in fact, not), which gives me even more motivation to put on sunscreen every day.

If you've got sunscreen on, your skin, instead of fighting off the incoming sun, can work on repair instead, so your skin will actually improve even if you wear only sunscreen and take no other antiaging measures.

ming his show tunes. Adam turned to me after the first few shots. "How do I look?"

"Um!" I said in numb horror at the sight of blood, my voice turning up in a desperate attempt to sound positive. I squeaked out an entirely unconvincing "You look great!" Collagen may be good for something, but it is very bloody, and then there's the whole mad cow thing.

"Really? You're not lying?"

"No, really!" I lied weakly.

TIP: With any sort of injection, get the topical anesthetic. It's messy and it takes about a half hour longer, but it's worth it.

Then it was my turn. I, being more wrinkled, got the Botox. Dr. Brandt did a few shots. Anyone who tells you it doesn't hurt or bandies about the word *discomfort* is a big fat liar. Again, Dr. Brandt did one side first (no neck, though; the thought is still just too horrifying).

"Oh, my God," Adam said in a hushed tone. "That's really unbelievable."

"What? What?" Did I look like a plastic version of myself, forever frozen into some awful grin? Was there blood everywhere?

"No, you look a thousand times younger," he said. "It's amazing."

I spent the next several hours waiting for the botulism to take over my body and paralyze me into my slow, torturous, and inevitable death, but it didn't happen.

The next day, in the bright, high-noon sun, I went swimming with Lisa, whom I'd told I was going for Botox several days before. "Notice anything different?" I asked, very pleased with myself.

She cocked her head to one side and looked at me. "Did you get your hair cut?" The invisible transformation: the best thing.

The kinds of people who are always horrified at women and vanity predictably have a great deal to say about Botox, usually involving Orwellian nightmares where women are no longer allowed to show emotions or aren't allowed to look their age, or where children can't properly attach to their frozen-faced parents. Mysteriously unlined actresses helpfully explain that *they* can't possibly get Botox because of their job (*acting!* not just sitting there looking glamorous!).

The thing is, like plastic surgery or makeup or even hair gel, Botox can be overdone—I would note that I've seen far more people who've visibly had too much plastic surgery than I have people who look as if they've had too much Botox. And it lasts for three or four months rather than being permanent, so there's always that.

Yes, it's sick to risk some awful but technically possible allergic reaction for the sake of looking a little better, but so is eating that toxic blowfish sushi that people love so much, or riding around on a motorcycle with your hair blowing in the wind, or any number of other sick and wrong things people do on a regular basis. We're women, so we just have to feel a little worse about it. Anyway.

Restylane, Collagen, Etc.

Botox erases wrinkles; these things fill an area. You can fill a wrinkle or a scar, or you can lessen the sagginess of, say, undereye bags by puffing up the spot right next to them. "Say there's a mountain," Dr. Brandt explains, always with the smile. "If you put a great big mountain of dirt next to the mountain, it doesn't look so tall."

An actress friend of mine was bitten in the face by a dog. She goes every three or four months for collagen injections, and I've never seen her looking as if she has any—*any*—sort of scar whatsoever. But collagen, as the crestfallen Adam will tell you, does not deliver the Heather Locklear effect. Restylane is similar but lasts longer. Bruising is much more common than with Botox. My friend Melanie got Restylane (Dr. Brandt, natch) and called me, horrified. "I look like I just lost a boxing match!" she wailed. But then she called me a week later, deliriously happy. And now she does, indeed, live the dream of looking precisely like herself ten years ago.

As with anything, it's possible to overdo filler injections; the results look like too much plastic surgery. The difference is, the plastic surgery is forever. Either way, perspective is all. I recently figured out the mystery behind all the overenhanced cheekbones: Why would someone choose such a thing? A dermatologist was speaking about fillers at an event; I was transfixed and horrified by the enormity of her cheekbones, which jutted out much the way a baboon's might, like sharp, hard shelves, clearly filled with too much filler. She began talking about the nasolabial fold, those lines that run from the end of your nose down around your mouth. "People used to try to inject the nasolabial fold," she explained (could there be a less appealing term than nasolabial fold, P.S.?). "It doesn't work. Those lines are cause by skin sagging down, so you've got to lift the skin above it—at the cheekbones." At last the mystery—*the why*—of the jutting cheekbones was solved, and it's the perfect example of cutting off your nose to spite your face, if you'll entertain that metaphor. In their desperation to completely rid the face of lines (all of the jutting-cheek celebrities have no nasolabial folds), these people (and their doctors) have lost sight of the overall goal, which would be to look better, not worse.

Facial and Peels

My powerful bias against the facial was probably formed when I did a story on them for *Vogue* and the beauty editor had me get nine of them in a week. My entire face ended up peeling off in sheets—yet my skin mysteriously wasn't red or irritated looking, so the peeling looked even more troubling, like some new form of leprosy. Because I wasn't red or otherwise injured, people stopped themselves before they blurted out, "Oh God, what happened to you?" and instead observed in silent, perplexed horror.

But the final facial improbably cured everything: I was scheduled to go to Georgette Klinger, and I called to ask whether I might just do the interview and not the facial, because my skin was so traumatized. Oh no, they said, Ms. Klinger will do the facial herself.

Ms. Klinger, it turned out, was a very fragile but still very beautiful ninety-something in a proper, stunning black Chanel suit, her white hair floating in a fabulous coif. She sat above the whole facial proceedings and made pronouncements (she was clearly too frail to do the actual treatment herself), which the aesthetician carried out. Ms. Klinger dictated layer upon layer of serums, liquids, and creams in an ever so certain order, and two hours later my skin was completely back to normal.

That's the thing about a facial. It absolutely depends on the person doing it. It's not the miracle products they claim it is, and it's not their special method; it's *them.* Some people are brilliant psychics; some people are brilliant politicians; some people are brilliant facialists. Dermatologists will say, diplomatically, that if facials relax you (as if!), go ahead, they're not going to hurt you. But if you get a facial from Sonya Dakar in Los Angeles, you walk out looking absolutely incredible. The first time I got one (she was in New York), I went back to the office literally without a speck of makeup on my face. I looked fantastic. Similarly, my friend Jennifer got a facial from Ole Henriksen in Los Angeles, and afterward he dragged her out into the parking lot, into the high-noon sun, and flashed his mirror at her there. Her wrinkles, her pores—everything was gone, and in its place was the smoothest, glowiest skin. In both cases, the effects wore off after a few days, but no one will ever convince me that *that* sort of facial isn't doing *something.*

On the other hand, there's a woman in New York for whom celebs literally line up to pay $500 for a facial, whom everyone in my department raved about. So we decided to do a story. "Take a model and have her get three facials," I said. "We'll do a before and after."

The film in my hand, I marched into Kim France's office. "Here are the shots of the model before and after the facials," I said, pulling them out. The two pictures were identical.

"There's no difference," she said, mystified.

"So it's proof, then. Facials don't really work!" I declared triumphantly.

"How much did we pay for all of this?" she asked.

I think the facial is most useful right before a big night out (as long as you've had the exact same facial from the exact

Face Cream Ingredients and Pascal's Wager

You know the "it doesn't hurt and it sure could help" reason to believe in God? The upside (going to heaven and avoiding hell) versus the downside (a little time spent being faithful, perhaps to no avail) being so lopsided that you might as well go for it? It works with skin care, too. And these ingredients do help.

- Retinol. Fantastic. It's what's in Retin-A, except not as strong.
- Alpha hydroxy acids (AHAs). Like retinol, they exfoliate and smooth the skin. As with retinol, the potency varies tremendously—there are products for people who get irritated at the tiniest percentage of AHA or retinol, and there are ones for Faces of Steel people (I fall into this camp), who feel that nothing short of H_2SO_4 is going to make them look better. As far as the zillions of companion products (cleansers, toners, etc.) that they impregnate with the miracle retinol or AHA to work in concert with the main-event cream or serum, this is what I'll say: They can't hurt, except perhaps in the pocketbook.
- Vitamin C. People debate its efficacy all the time and are always arguing over whether a certain brand goes bad too fast, is unstable, etc. The thing is, people who try it always come back for more. It makes your skin sort of brighter, sort of clearer. Even men—who are generally much less trusting of products than women—love it. The machismo central Playboy used to come in demanding only two things: an AHA sunscreen cream from Ralph Lauren and vitamin C serum. "It work!" he would say in his cheerful, near incomprehensible, Gallic way. "You write about, no?"
- Anti-inflammatories. The whole theory about inflammation causing disease and aging makes an enormous amount of sense to me. My sunscreen has anti-inflammatories even.

Still More Ingredients

- Antioxidants. In general—green tea, white tea, pomegranate extract, vitamin E, all of it—I take the Pascal's wager approach. They help in theory, at the very least.
- The ingredient I'm not willing to wager on is anything in any way suggestive of mad cow disease association. Your bovine collagen/placenta/embryo-type ingredients could be the fountain of youth, and I still wouldn't go for it. Besides the terrifying aspect, it's all just too foul.

same person on a different occasion and you emerged glowing rather than mottled).

People with great skin always attribute it to something—I've heard everything, from Ivory soap to regular facials to sleeping only on the back of your head (this last one always gives me pause, and I think about it often, but I can't make it happen)—rather than just thanking God for their luck of the genetic draw. The point is, don't assume that so-and-so's once-a-month facials are the reason she looks so great.

Peels, depending on how strong they are, can make a more permanent difference. A deep peel is a bloody endeavor that requires recovery time and can leave your skin utterly pigmentless—hence the deathly pall of some older yet smooth-skinned women.

I once went for media training and ended up in the apartment of just such a woman. She was very thin, which, along with the pallor, gave her a decidedly ghostly air; she looked about fifty but was eerily lineless. Then she shook my hand,

and *her* hands—along with being startlingly large—revealed an age that was closer to eighty. Both the hard evidence of her true age and the fact that she'd endured this horrific peel hung in the air between us like an enormous, moaning elephant. Whatever desperate measures you may find me taking in my later years, a deep peel/dermabrasion will not be happening.

Lighter peels—with varying concentrations of acids or with microcrystals shot from sort of a reverse vacuum—can make a less marked but still significant improvement in your skin. Like the AHAs and retinols, they speed up exfoliation, and like the AHAs and retinols, they vary widely in quality and concentration; you just have to experiment. Go somewhere (derm or spa) where you know people have gone before and lived to tell the tale.

Similarly, light dermabrasion—where they shoot aluminum crystals at your skin—works to some noticeable degree and involves no downtime or undue risk. It's often called "crystal clearing" at spas, "microdermabrasion" at doctors' offices. You can now buy creams that contain the aluminum crystals; you scrub your face with them in a way that's not painful but to me is deeply grating, like nails on a chalkboard. You emerge glowing—ever so imperceptibly—but I can't help obsessing

Antiager Tip

Just getting your face a little wet increases the efficacy of both retinol and AHAs (for some people, to the point that a perfectly good product for them is rendered far too irritating; for others, making them younger faster).

over the word *aluminum*, with all the nonstick pans and the Alzheimer's.

Lasers

I *once* got a bikini wax. I've had natural childbirth twice and endured several other episodes of significant pain in my life, and all I can say is, never again. How most women can march in once or twice a month for it is completely beyond me, and the people who do it to themselves are even more incredible. And the worst is, they don't have to: Laser hair removal hurts about one-eightieth the amount that waxing does, and it gets rid of most of your hair forever! It's genius! It takes five minutes! Even if you have to go back in for a touch-up, who cares? Anything's better (even Nair, I'll say it right here) than a wax.

But lasers have turned out to be good for other things, too. I once went to the office of a famous dermatologist who was helping a skin care company launch its latest creams. (Because of all the plastic surgery and Botox and dermatologist skin care lines, every big company now employs a dermatologist to tout its products and, depending on the situation, give advice.) I had been to *my* dermatologist the day before and had gotten a Gentle Waves laser treatment, an entirely painless procedure where you put on goggles and they flash a light at you for forty seconds.

After the presentation, the skin care people told me I could go for a free session with the famous dermatologist. "Oh, that's okay," I told them. "I was just at the dermatologist yesterday."

The famous dermatologist looked at me. "You got Gentle Waves, didn't you," she said. "Your skin looks great. It's got that glow."

Another famous dermatologist told me she got her Gentle Waves machine when she went to a conference and saw three doctors she'd interned with. "Their skin looked fantastic," she said. "They said it was the Gentle Waves."

Lasers have suffered terribly from the awful names their manufacturers give them (nyg-this, yag-that, ablative whatever, it all sounds terrifying), and like peels, they encompass a vast variety of treatments, levels of severity, and results.

Laser resurfacing is like dermabrasion, involving pain and recovery time, and can really do a number on your wrinkles. The risks include being noticeably red faced for six months, infection, and all the rest. You'd want to be very serious about antiaging before resorting to this.

Then there are lasers to zap broken capillaries and age spots, and while these involve a little pain (as in . . . *zap!*), they work, have few risks, and take all of five minutes, typically.

Then there are lasers like Gentle Waves, for general revivification—they work mostly to stimulate collagen production in your skin. Some require prescription-level pain medication and reportedly take ten years off your face (tightening the jawline, for instance, which is something you'd otherwise need plastic surgery for, or at least liposuction; either way, ouch); others are milder and promise to decrease wrinkles, pore size, and sagginess over time. Do they work? Well, as with face creams, it's anybody's guess.

New Age Mumbo Jumbo

Just as your average old person who's spent years smoking generally looks like hell (I once took a continuing ed creative writing course at the University of New Mexico in Albuquerque; the combination of sun and smoking had rendered some of the older students into Yoda-like specters who croaked out their poems and short stories from faces that looked like the desiccated sandals of, say, Jesus, were someone to recover them from an archaeological dig in the Holy Land), I have to report that your average old yoga person looks like a million bucks. There are exceptions to both rules, but it's just something I've observed. At the Ashram, the aforementioned torture camp/yoga-and-hiking spa in Los Angeles, the genuinely crazy people who ran it and exhorted us to hike farther and faster in the zillion-degree heat, and not eat so we could be more like the Breath-Airians, did look fabulous despite advanced age. By fabulous, I don't mean just a great body, either, which the major yoga practitioner always has in spades; I mean a practically lineless, unsagging, youthful face.

The most important thing about all of it is that even if your antiaging strategy actually succeeds in making you look younger, you will still look like you, just younger, and if you're dissatisfied with that to begin with, you're not going to be any happier. And then you could end up like one of those crazy people who keep going back and back and back to the plastic surgeon, and *Allure* will ask you to write an embarrassing essay, and God knows what it'll say on your epitaph.

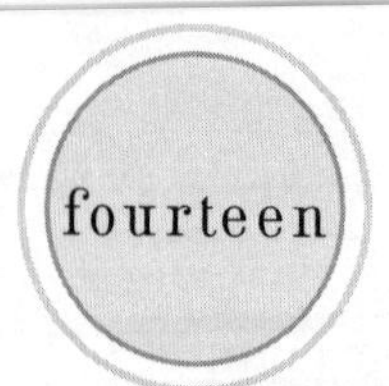

fourteen

The Dumbest Career Move Ever

All of a sudden, I'd been at *Elle* for six years, and they'd fired most of the people I loved and respected; I knew my time there would be up soon, and I knew, from having watched so many tragic *Elle* endings, that it wouldn't be pretty. They hired a new French art director, whom I loathed and who loathed me back. He was freckled and do-ragged and sexist and prone to bombastic outbursts that came very close to being physical. Very in-your-face: "BUT I AM A FAMOUS ART DIRECTOR! YOUUUU LEESTEN TO MEEEE!" We had several epic screaming matches.

On top of that, there was a new French editorial overseer—sort of a replacement for the now deposed Eminence Grise—whom I loathed and who loathed me back. It was also 1999, and everyone and their brother was jumping ship for the Internet, and Beautyscene.com, an e-commerce beauty site, called me and asked me to run their online magazine.

For a few short weeks in September or October 1999, every very rich or even vaguely rich person could not wait to get his or her hands on an upcoming IPO. "Internet!" they'd say. "Internet! And beauty products! Great idea!" It looked as though impossible riches were to be made and that at last I, too, could have the money *and* the glamour.

"You are leaving?" the new French overseer blinked in amazement. "You have been . . . so very lucky . . . at *Elle.*"

"*Elle*"—I glared back at him—"has been lucky to have me."

Was I crazy to leave it all? The section I'd stayed up all those nights building into something that I, the readers, and my superiors all liked? My column? My relationships with other writers, editors, advertisers, art people, photographers? Certainly plenty of it was going to translate—somehow, hopefully. It was a difficult decision. Made worse, for me, by the after-school-special feeling I have that contemplating any sort of change now necessitates making said change. "Change is good" is always the moral of the story, isn't it? Moving on, it seemed, was the only adult option.

I envisioned my departure as a jump, Nestea-like, into a deep, cerulean pool. A pool like the one in the old Chanel commercial. "Welcome to the new economy!" e-mailed an already rich Microsoft operative.

I jumped. Practically the next day, I was on a plane to Northern California, Internet ground zero—and my hometown. I was there before the nerds had ever discovered running shoes, where computers took up entire rooms in buildings made of cinder blocks. Stacks of ugly manila cards with tiny rectangular punch holes. Cheap little suburban office parks with tinted windows. Before it meant more money than anyone could ever conceive of. Pre-Jobs. Pre-Gates. Pre-Po (Bronson). Pre-IPO. I knew these people, and I spoke their language, or so I thought.

Menlo Park, California: home of my mother, and home of the Money People. I figured I was serving as a sort of window dressing—my various bosses would discuss whatever it was you discussed with Money People, and I would sort of authenticate things, being from a big magazine and all. As we sped up Route 280 from San Francisco, almost to the Sand Hill Road exit that I knew so well, the owner—a tiny, body-building-crazed man in an odd waistcoat (which he later explained, with great pride, had been bought at an auction and had originally been one of Elton John's own bespoke morning coats)—turned around and addressed us in the backseat. "So," he said, "what are we going to say to these people?" I thought he meant, "Exactly how am I going to phrase things this time?" or "Which of our many good points should be brought up first?" We'll call him Tiny Gym Rat.

About ten minutes into the actual meeting, the running-shoe-clad Money Person turned to me rather disdainfully and sighed. "So what," he said, "is your big idea?" I turned back toward my new superiors, cueing them to start their pitch. They looked back at me with big open faces, expectant smiles.

I have no idea what I said. I talked beauty as I've never talked beauty before; I prophesied; I gesticulated wildly. The Money Person noted that his wife liked spas, so I had lots to say about mud wraps and facials. We didn't get the money.

Beyond the money-getting part, the rest of my job, at first, did not seem so terribly different from magazines: The big idea behind Beautyscene.com was a combination of content and commerce, which made so much sense at the time.

With the Internet, you could change things every day, every hour, if you liked, the way a newspaper might. I was excited about covering subjects—things like how to deal with acne, say, or wrinkles—that are difficult to address fully in a magazine, because of the space they take up. I liked the instant feedback—that you could see how many people read a given article and how long they spent reading it before they clicked off.

The biggest challenge revolved around the pictures. If you're going to buy something like a new lipstick, you want to know what it looks like. When I arrived at Beautyscene, the pictures (for both content and commerce) were the size of ant droppings. And unlovely ant droppings they were—except in the eyes of their creators, the Tech People. "Oh no," they said. "The pictures cannot be bigger."

Almost anything I wanted to change was impossible. It increased downloading times, or the Internet "just doesn't work that way."

"Well, we can't change that today, the Bombay Team is in charge of that." Well, I'd say, call up the Bombay Team. I'm thinking "Bombay" is "B," as in, "The Alpha Team is in charge of this, and the Bombay Team is in charge of that." As it turned out, the Bombay Team was actually a team somewhere in Bombay, and no one had their number.

I needed an art director. I called up my old friend Adam and managed (to my great shame later on) to steal him away from the Prada/Versace/Narciso Rodriguez/Kate Moss job he was busy making zillions at. He thought the same thing I did: In short order, we'd be rich pioneers. "We'll be the Fred and Ginger of the Internet," he said.

The Tech People thought Adam was ridiculous. "That orange dot you've designed is just a bad color for the Web," they'd say. "We think blue is much nicer. And no, we can't make the pictures bigger."

Finally, Adam and I hired our own Tech Person. "Can you

make the pictures bigger?" we demanded as soon as the Tech Person arrived.

"Oh yes," he said. "I'll do it this afternoon." The Tech People had simply been stonewalling—for months on end.

There were also layers and layers of management, most of them former or current boyfriends of Tiny Gym Rat. "My lucky jacket!" he would say, getting ready for yet another try-to-drum-up-cash meeting.

By far the best money meeting was held deep in New Jersey, at the bottom of a very ornate restaurant called Vinnie's or Sal's or something. We presented our big idea to about twenty brokers, each one straight out of *The Sopranos*, each one representing "individual investors" (one of whom, a resident of Switzerland, was looking to spend about $60 million).

"The Internet!" boomed the hirsute Mr. $60 Million Client after we'd finished our presentation. He squeezed a fat lemon wedge over his veal cutlet. "Beauty products! This is gonna be huge—you know, especially with all the old people." Not exactly our market (the elderly, not renowned for their e-savvy), but okay. "They get that disease, you know, where they're afraid to go out of their houses?" he continued, elbowing a shiny-suited compatriot. "That disease, you know, Freddie, what's it called? My friend's wife had it—what is that thing? It's tragic, something happens to your mind—mostly it's the old people, the elderly—they can't leave their homes, it's like an, an irrational fear . . . homophobia! These people, they get homophobia and they can't leave the house. It's so sad. But plenty of 'em have lots of money. And they still want beauty products, but they can't go out to get 'em!"

I nodded my head enthusiastically and went on to detail the many other reasons why they should allocate huge portions of their clients' fortunes to invest in our site. I slowly realized, post espresso, as I was shaking hands and distributing my card, that were these men to invest, and were that investment to not pan out for some reason, they'd be left holding . . . a business card with my name on it.

We didn't get the money—we didn't get any money, it turned out. But the people running the company didn't mention that to us until December 24, the day before Christmas and three weeks after I'd hired a team of writers, photographers, and, of course, one of my best friends. Tiny Gym Rat announced (via conference call) that he was sorry, we weren't going to be getting our paychecks that week, because they were out of money, and they'd been out of money for a long time, and the cabal of ex-boyfriends had paid only those bills that might, left unpaid, red-flag the fact that they were completely broke and essentially stealing goods and services from all sorts of companies and individuals.

There was the photographer who'd shot about $40,000 worth of pictures for us—who happened to be married to the beauty editor of *Vogue*—who'd gone unpaid, for instance. Career suicide for Adam and me, since the photographer was also repped by the most important photography/illustration agent in all of New York. Adam insisted on a conference call to San Francisco (Tiny Gym Rat had retreated to his mansion there and had been spitting out confused, seemingly drug-addled e-mails for several weeks). I didn't think it would do anything but agreed anyway. We started the conference call, Adam with his calming, soothing voice and the owner's shaking, amped-up one trading back and forth. "But you don't understand, I don't *have* any money to give you. . . ."

And then appeared the "I'll kill them all" Adam, the one he'd hinted at in the *The Accused* diner. He spoke through his teeth, he pounded his fists on the table, he threatened, he swore, and . . . he got the money. A personal check from hideous Tiny Gym Rat, one that did not bounce and that indeed saved our careers, at least for the moment.

We stuck it out while they weren't paying us, while Tiny Gym Rat was trying desperately to sell the company; it was no fun. You'd open the door into the expensive SoHo loft space with its groovy, creative workstations jeering at you every morning and feel like screaming, and the feeling would only intensify as the hours—spent quibbling with this person and then that one—ground slowly on. No, Can't, Sorry . . . It was all that, all the time, and it was interminably boring.

Adam and I had desks facing each other; the despair flicked back and forth between us like a worn-out tennis ball. Each day contained two highlights. First was lunch, where we ate vast quantities of egg whites scrambled with chili peppers, spied on Sarah Jessica Parker (who was often at the next table at the diner we favored), and played "Would You Rather?"—a game in which you choose between two horrible scenarios (typically sexual, always involving unappealing co-workers).

Then there was our 4:00 p.m. break at the juice store. There, the "Would You Rather?" continued apace as the organic but cute juice makers indulged our theories about what the best-tasting smoothies might contain. Mine was watermelon, lime, strawberry, and ginger; the "Would You Rather?" that defeated me invariably involved servicing one or another of our unappealing co-workers after he'd completed a half hour of jumping jacks on the roof of our building in the ninety-five-degree heat.

Adam preferred pineapple, wheatgrass, and banana. The "Would You Rather?" that got him was this: You've got an interview with Anna Wintour, and you must wear the Elton John waistcoat with the Tiny Gym Rat black muscle T-shirt and pleated black trousers underneath. Not only must you feature the waistcoat and bring it up in the conversation several times, but you must explain, in detail, how you bought it at auction, brag proudly about whom it once belonged to, etc. Even the most grotesque unappealing co-worker option always won over this one.

Scrambled egg whites, fruit smoothie, another day over, thank God. The air in the office smelled like Band-Aids, and it was tedious and awful.

I would go to the odd beauty event to keep up appearances—many cosmetics companies were unimpressed with the Internet at that point and thus unimpressed with me, their former darling; but there were still plenty of people interested in hawking something, or at least in convincing a warm body to fill a seat at their next lunch. Beautyscene.com still appeared successful—there were huge ads by a famous photographer with a famous model in practically every magazine on the planet and on buses and billboards, too (all unpaid for, it later turned out). I kept cranking out content; the site kept making sales. But to the people who counted, I was nobody, or close to it. It was nice, however, to have the obsequiousness dial turned dramatically down. People cared much less about whether I believed their cellulite-cream claims.

I helped the lame Beautyscene.comers sell the company to an oily investor. We immediately blackmailed ("I'm telling everything to *Women's Wear*!") the new guy into paying everyone's back salary, so it wasn't a total loss, but the air still smelled of failure and Band-Aids, and the whole thing was still a sinking ship of desperate, unhappy people.

Then, thank God, a big fashion company came along and snapped up Adam, reinstalling him into the world of actual glamour and zillions to which he was accustomed. And a few months later, my old friend Kim France (she had been one of the original *Elle* operatives who tolerated my red lipstick experiments) gave me a call. She'd created a new magazine for Condé Nast called *Lucky*, and she needed a beauty editor.

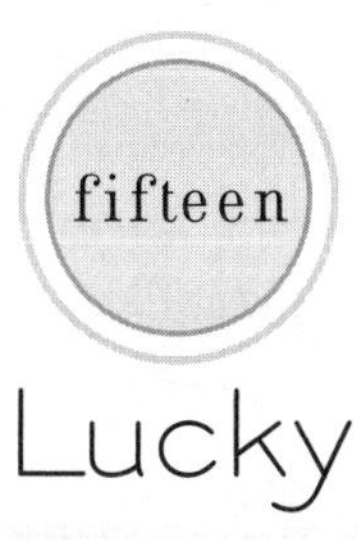

fifteen

Lucky

All predictable puns aside, I couldn't have been luckier. Why they were willing to take a chance on me, I'll never know, but *Lucky* certainly saved my career.

While I am glad, in retrospect, that I left *Elle* and tried the nightmare Internet and learned that lesson, I no longer feel that change and moving on up is necessarily always the better option. *Lucky* has been a relief, a challenge, and a pleasure.

My first day at *Lucky*, halfway through the afternoon, James Truman, Condé Nast's then editorial director, and Si Newhouse, its owner, suddenly appeared in my office. I of course took their appearance to mean something about my relative importance, but I think they were actually reviewing the office design, and mine was an example of one of the new, private-but-not-exactly-private offices.

"Oh, hello, Jean," Mr. Truman said jovially. "Meet Mr. Newhouse. Si, this is our new beauty director for *Lucky*."

They continued glancing around the room, noting wall heights and such. "Now, which of the dot-coms were you working for?" asked Mr. Truman. A casual and reasonable question, except for the multipage Beautyscene.com advertising spreads I suddenly remembered seeing plastered all over the September *Vogue*, *Glamour*, and *Vanity Fair* (all

Condé Nast magazines) the previous year; they had looked fantastic. I remembered how impressed I was at how much money Beautyscene must've had to buy all those ads.

"Uh . . . um . . . Beautyscene.com," I squeaked, trying to sound casual and upbeat.

Mr. Newhouse folded his arms and the two of them regarded me with expressions that balanced between quizzical and cold. And out they stalked.

I was amazed not to have been fired then and there. I was also, as I adjusted to my new job and began noticing the people around me, amazed to have made it through the hiring process. Everyone makes jokes about Condé Nast and its quest for physical perfection in its employees. Certainly a cursory glance at any of the lines in the Frank Gehry–designed cafeteria (the terrazzo floors had to be reworked so as not to catch stiletto heels, to protect the fabulous from upset and injury) at lunchtime will raise suspicions that the genes for beauty and appearance-consciousness are cross-linked with those for magazine aptitude. It's sort of an all-business version of the Playboy mansion or one of those islands where James Bond and Captain Kirk are always landing, populated exclusively by beautiful and frightening women.

There are the stunningly gorgeous people, the plain pretty, the acceptably groomed (most days I manage to fit into this category), and, last, the not attractive *and* unacceptably groomed. Counterintuitively, you actually cut quite a swath if you're a member of the final group, because it means you're either (1) wildly talented and thus indispensable, or (2) willing to do a job everyone else hates and thus indispensable. As close to tenure as it gets at Condé Nast, anyway.

I have overheard the words "Does that girl work at *Vogue* or

A Really Good Coco Chanel Quote

Are you as tired of bons mots from Mme. Chanel as I? Nonetheless, this saved my life one day as I was riding up the Condé Nast elevator and realized midascent that I was due to make a speech to the sales department in two minutes. The speech was supposed to be in response to the several copycat magazines that have emerged as *Lucky* has become more successful.

Condé Nast has several of those elevator televisions that flash stock quotes and weather predictions so everyone has something to look at; when there's no good news to speak of, it churns out quotes.

"In order to be indispensable, you must be different," flashed the elevator TV. Brilliant, no?

Vanity Fair?" (read: she's really hot) while standing in the lunch line. But getting prospective employees past the *Lucky* operatives involves highlighting the reverse qualifications. If Kim uses the word *perfect* to describe someone, it's not a good sign. "She's overperfect!" Kim once said of an impeccable, extremely fashiony staff member, who, incidentally, ejected herself early on. (There are plenty of superhot gals at *Lucky*, don't get me wrong, by perfect I mean that smug, overly groomed, tucked-and-folded-scarf thing that some pretty girls feel enhances their attractiveness.)

At *Lucky*, the usual fashion magazine pecking order is all out of whack. Most notably, the fashion department is not mean. They're not constantly firing one another and sniping at non-fashion-department members in the hallways. Temper tantrums are rare. Screaming is rare, and cowering is rare.

Everyone (the whole staff, not just the fashion department) generally gets along.

It's why people like the magazine, I think, in the end. It's about having your own style and appreciating your friends' styles. One of the most popular pages is "Four Girls, One . . . [circle skirt or pair of stiletto boots or some such]," where four real girls show what they'd wear a particular item with. The interesting part is how different they are—as it is in real life.

When you're leafing through just about any other magazine, you come to a fashion story, and you look at the model, and maybe she's too skinny or she looks nothing like you, or whatever. You look at the clothes, and maybe you hate the way they're styled, or you'd never wear that, or they're too expensive. If any of these things is the case, you move on to the next story, because there's nothing there for you. *Lucky* is less about the model and more about the many options on the page facing her. The options are there for *you* to choose from; it's about you. You don't have to love the model or even the way we styled her.

We ask makeup artists how to do a look in real life, rather than how they did it at Whoever-Fabulous's runway show. And we make them tell you their favorite products, and where to get them.

But if I felt shunned by the usual PR sycophants during the dot-com nightmare, it was nothing compared with how it felt when I started at *Lucky*. People simply hated us. "It's a catalog!" was the usual complaint. Never mind the Condé Nast pedigree. "Who needs another magazine? Another catalog, for that matter?" No tickets for fashion shows, no big press trips to fancy locales, and very few ads at first.

I felt the industry's initial contempt and disgust most

acutely when my publisher and I went on our most important business trip of the year, otherwise known as the CTFA. CTFA stands for Cosmetic, Toiletry, and Fragrance Association. Their annual convention is every March in sunny but not-so-fabulous Boca Raton, Florida. The suppliers to the beauty companies are there, the beauty companies are there, and all the magazine salespeople go to see the beauty company people. Never mind that the vast majority of the attendees are all based in New York and might just as well meet with one another there.

Everyone stays at a hotel called the Boca Raton Resort and Club; each company—magazine, beauty company, etc.—is assigned a cabana. "Cabana" sounds glamorous but is actually a small outdoor cement room in a sort of apartment complex arrangement near the resort's pools. You hop from cabana to cabana to have meetings with everyone, and the schedule is relentless: 8:30 a.m., 9:00 a.m., 9:30 a.m.—like that, all day, for two and a half days.

The magazine salespeople bring editors with them to explain the vision behind the beauty pages. You talk about what makes your magazine different from all others, what your readers respond to best, what portion of the magazine is devoted to beauty editorial, if there are any changes or new initiatives on the horizon.

At the CTFA, the tables are turned, for the most part, with the editors doing the talking and the cosmetics company exectives doing the listening. Presenting your editorial vision while squished on the edge of a communal chaise lounge, squinting into the fierce Florida sun while your competitors hover nearby, sharpening their knives, is stressful. Each magazine tries to outdo the other, but because we're all sitting by the pool, the presentations can't be terribly elaborate. PowerPoint, thank God, is out of the question. And the teen magazines throw free concerts (boy bands are big) in the middle of everything, making it impossible to hear what anyone is saying.

I am always incredibly grateful for those meetings where they've got products to tell me about, so I can sink back into the role I'm most comfortable in. "We've got a new lipstick!" the PR woman will say, and I'll want to kiss her.

The look is reminiscent of an especially low beach scene in Ibiza, where the gnarliest, most wizened interlopers stroll blithely about in the tiniest bikinis and banana hammocks. Except at the CTFA they're wearing them while they're presenting their products and complaining about your magazine. Once, at *Elle*, we had to make a presentation to a powerful cosmetics executive as the sun set—he had chosen to meet us at the outdoor bar instead of a cabana and appeared to have already consumed about fifteen cocktails before we got there. Overweight and sixtyish, he wore a small, faded pair of red trunks and that was it; his skin was leathery and oiled to a high sheen. I began my spiel about my editorial philosophy; he pulled out his cigar and regarded me as if I were auditioning to become his private lap dancer. "Honey," he slurred, "all I care about's the CPM [cost per million; magazines with enormous circulations like *Cosmo* and *Glamour* have a high CPM, and fancier niche magazines like *Elle* and *W* do not]. I don' care what the magazine *says*— " And he fell out of his chair.

My publisher would wear his bathing suit and recline in the sun, smoking a cigar; his archrival, Ron Galotti, the publisher of *Vogue* (otherwise known as Mr. Big from *Sex and the City*), did the same directly across the way, each pretending not to see the other. The president of our company dropped by one day (in a white Rolls-Royce, natch), also smoking a cigar, outfitted in a skimpy pair of Dolphin shorts.

The then beauty editor at *Vogue* (with whom I had the pact about each of us calling the other so we never ran the same products) and I made another pact that no matter how many people turned up in bikinis and inappropriate shorts, we would both wear clothing—actual, even businesslike clothing—to the end.

At *Lucky*, so far, no one has tried to wear a bathing suit. Our publisher is that sort of powerful woman who exudes a formality that seems the natural consequence of having been gorgeous all her life. At her most casual, she'll wear a sundress, but it'll be by Chanel and there'll be a cardigan to go with it.

At the base of it, bathing suits or no, we stay in a glamorous hotel and soak up the sun for a few days. I think I simply wasn't cut out for conventions. Who is, really?

The first year of *Lucky*, our fellow CTFA conventioneers hated us so much, they wouldn't even meet with us. We could've worn diamanté thongs and not gotten any attention. My publisher and I spent most of our time at the hotel restaurant, casting about for familiar faces and making small talk. "Um, it's great to see you," people I'd once thought of as friendly would say, wincing as they rushed by. The final afternoon, we agreed that we couldn't take it anymore and retired to our respective rooms. I called in to work, called all my friends to no avail, and ended up lurching tragically around the room, chewing Toblerone bars from the minibar (even the finest chocolate turns waxy and cardboard flavored when you're bored and/or deeply shamed), making myself sick, and thinking back to the good old days at Beautyscene.com, where at least people liked the concept.

I felt so miserable, in fact, that I eventually occupied myself by scribbling rants on the back of some press release for anti-aging cream; the result, a total rip-off of the brilliant fiction writer Daniel Orozco, does take some license with the facts, but you get the basic idea:

This is an Information Packet. It contains a directory of the names, titles, and corporate affiliations of your fellow attendees. This is an updated directory: The directory you received in the mail may not have been complete. If your name is on the list in the directory, then I will be able to give you your own Information Packet. If your name is not on the list, you will first have to see Donna at the Welcome Desk. Donna is the one with the carnation pink lipstick near the bird of paradise flower arrangement on the left side of the Welcome Desk. When she smiles, you'll notice she's missing a few teeth. Don't say anything. Donna practices self-hypnosis for pain management, so if you see her looking a little dreamy, just wait. Your charge will be $956.43, which includes a $50 late-registration fee. Yes, we take credit cards; Diner's Club is preferred.

The $956.43 will not get your name onto the list—this is only for prepaid attendees—but it will officially register your name and company affiliation with us, and I will be able to give you your own Information Packet. Without your Information Packet, you may not attend any of the sessions and will be asked to leave.

In the Information Packet you will find your laminated ID badge, which you must wear at all times. If this is your first time here, there will be a red sticker on your badge; this will admit you to the First Timer's Reception, which will be at seven o'clock in the Galleon Room. Please do not attend the First Timer's Reception if your badge does not have a red sticker.

Also in your Information Packet you will find a yellow or a pink ticket for the Look Great, Feel Fabulous! Banquet Gala. If you do not find a yellow or pink ticket in your packet, you may have registered incorrectly, or you may not be prepaid. You will not be admitted to the LGFF! Gala without a ticket. If you have a yellow ticket, you have been designated Table Captain for your table and will need to return to this desk tomorrow to register. Table captains must register their tables or they will not be on the LGFF! Gala list. We use this list to arrange tables for the banquet; if your table is not on it, none of your guests will be seated. If your Information Packet contains a pink ticket, you do not need to register tomorrow, but let's hope your Table Captain does. Check with your Table Captain for any last-minute details.

Additional tables for the LGFF! Gala are available for $5,000 per table. While individuals may make private donations of any amount they wish to LGFF!, individual contributions will not admit you to the gala: You must be assigned to a table and present your pink ticket or a validated Table Captain's registration at the door of the event.

You may distribute authorized promotional materials in designated areas. Attendees found distributing unauthorized promotional materials or hosting unauthorized events will be asked to leave. If your event is not on the schedule, it is not authorized. Please do not ask me to put any additional events on the schedule; our events have been carefully planned and prepaid, and we cannot accommodate additional requests. You may hear Larry Schine boasting that we have scheduled events for him and his company at the last minute, because he is on the board of directors. He makes these boasts every year and they are not true and you should ignore them. Elaine Brown, Larry's long-suffering secretary back in Houston, actually arranges their company events here at least eight months in advance, sometimes more. Elaine Brown has never, in all her years, attended this conference (so I have never personally met her), but she is very dedicated and arranges Larry's events early on to avoid any problems.

You will notice a sheet in your packet about the Steering Committee Cocktail Hour, which you may notice does not appear on your schedule. This does not mean it is an unauthorized event. The SCCH is not on the schedule because of an oversight in our office. One of my assistants, DeeDee Vanderbyle, neglected to enter it onto the events schedule, and when the preliminary schedule was sent to the board for approval, it was signed off on anyway—no one caught the error—and the schedule was sent on to the printer. DeeDee Vanderbyle was going through a nasty child custody case and may have been distracted when she drew up the preliminary schedule (of course this is not your concern), and she has been asked to leave.

I will be going over all of this information again (except, naturally, the incident with Ms. Vanderbyle and our organization) at the First Timer's Reception. If you have a red sticker on your ID badge, please feel welcome to attend. There will be an open bar with cocktails, beer, and wine; dress is casual.

○

Back in New York, it wasn't any better—for a while. But much as the industry hated our concept, readers started to love it; they showed their love by subscribing in record numbers and buying truckloads of whatever items we put in the magazine. The best instance of this was a picture of a stylist we ran. The stylist had made a watch out of a regular old Timex and the ribbed elastic band off some Gucci luggage (the band was that distinctive red, green, and brown Gucci stripe). Though you could barely even see the "Gucci watch" in the picture, Gucci was nonetheless overwhelmed with calls from potential customers demanding to know where they could buy the watch; they were so insistent, in fact, that Gucci ended up making the watch.

We'd run some obscure, not-new nail polish, and it'd sell out across the country. I remember being thirteen and reading *Seventeen,* poring over the fashion credits, and wondering, desperately, what Reminiscence and Agnes B. were, and where they were located, and whether someone like me could ever hope to afford or even find the item on the pages. Fantasy is great and everything, but at *Lucky* the fantasy can become reality in short order, which, as it turns out, is deeply satisfying to many.

The fantasy of availability is itself incredibly powerful. The Garnet Hill catalog, which rarely has anything that appeals to me, gets hours of my undivided attention whenever it arrives in my mailbox. Ditto, insanely, the Bliss catalog, which is full of nothing but . . . the beauty products I already have sitting in my office. It doesn't matter; I study it as though my life depends on it.

It's funny: When I used to tell people I worked at *Elle,* they were very impressed. "Oh," they'd say, regarding me with a new respect, "that's a really big magazine!" When I tell people I work at *Lucky,* they're not quite as impressed in that "wow, you're so important" way. Instead it's, "Oh my God: MY magazine! I discovered it! I love it! You work there?"

By the time a year had passed and we were back at the soul-crushing go-rounds of CTFA, we had plenty of meetings. Everyone—the PR people, the advertising people, other magazines—wanted to be the next *Lucky*, to look like *Lucky*, to capture the *Lucky* reader. . . .

Lucky Girls

So I leave the house every morning and I come into work and I do feel lucky, there's no two ways about it. They let me create my section of the magazine without a great deal of intervention or hemming and hawing. They like new ideas. There's free coffee. People are not constantly torturing one another.

We do have to get through a good deal more product than I had to at *Elle*. People always ask me, How do you decide which beauty products to put in the magazine? It is very much like shopping. There are brilliant, glittering new items that, toylike, are impossible not to pick up and fool with, be charmed by, and want to possess forever. There's the thing with results that can't be denied, no matter how hideous it looks. Most of all, there's that thing your girlfriend told you was fantastic. *That's* the thing everyone wants to know.

There's a list of products we have to be careful about running—because we've run them too many times between us raving about them, and the real women we feature raving about them, and makeup artists and hair stylists raving about them. It's frustrating, because I'd like to say in every issue that

Laura Mercier's concealer is the best, just in case I missed someone the previous month.

While no item is ever "out" or "over" or "not" in *Lucky* (as in "hot: not" stories), Kim is forever banning overused words—we ripped through "bohemian" in the first year; "glamorous" and "amazing" are currently on the endangered list. "Fashionista" has been banned from the start.

Kim is not about a fashionista. She's an outsider to fashion, and that's why we've been a success. She doesn't accept something automatically because the fashion people say so; she demands to know in what situation you'd actually wear something like that. She's got access to every Prada and Carolina Herrera and Michael Kors in the world, and while she does wear them, the main event always seems to be some quirky thing she picked up in some out-of-the-way shop in Brooklyn.

Kim is smart smart smart and beautiful and successful (I know, kissing up to the boss, but it's true), but she doesn't look at the world from that vantage point. As far as she sees it, she's still trying to keep up, trying to figure it out, get it right. She's been there, and she remembers. She's impatient with the slick answer, the predigested tidbit—you'd think, We're working for *Lucky*, our articles are barely longer than captions, why wouldn't we be the kings of slick answers? But she has no time for them, so we search for something else, and it ends up being better.

I want to kill her when she says, "But I've seen that story a thousand times!" or, "Explain this to me!" or, "Banned word!" But she knows what she's doing, and I've learned a lot.

I realize that I, too, have banned words. *Tresses* and *locks* are my most hated. I'm not for a word people don't ever use in real life. *Frock* falls into this category as well. The reason you see these words in magazines at all is because overzealous copy editors will do anything to avoid repeating a word on the same page, so they force people to come up with these inanities instead of simply saying *hair* twice. I think a repeat is far more acceptable than a word no one uses. My test for any piece of writing I'm involved with is known around the office as the "Say this aloud to your smartest friend" test. Would the friend look at you as if you were crazy? Don't write it that way, then.

Many magazines—like anything else, books, TV shows, movies—dumb things down for their readers. And they shorten the articles to the point of meaninglessness. *Lucky* has the shortest articles imaginable, but we try our best to fight the short-article magazine diseases: alliteration ("Ten top ways to tame your tresses!"), leaving out all information except the obvious ("Substitute fruits and veggies for junk food!" "Go to a reputable doctor!" "No thong bikinis at the office picnic!"), and general pigheadedness ("Your Go-to Sexual Fantasies!").

We run lots of real people (instead of celebrities) raving about their favorite products. There are plenty of great celeb magazines, so we felt, why reinvent the wheel for the ninetieth time? (We do put celebrities on our cover, because, it turns out, you can't sell a magazine without a celebrity on the cover these days; we try to stick to their favorite places and things to shop for as subject matter, however, rather than their movies and boyfriends.)

As a result, we're always on the hunt for hot real girls to photograph. If someone's going to a supercool club, we'll remind them on the way out the door to be on the lookout for good-looking girls; it's very *Maxim.* "OmigodImetthecutest-girl!" is a common, welcome, and triumphant refrain.

Counterintuitively, we have to reject a lot of people at *Lucky*. Not PR, "no thanks, we don't cover plastic surgery" (my very favorite thing about working for *Lucky*, P.S.) rejection, real-person rejection. People look at *Vogue* or *Elle* and they know it's a fantasy. They understand that the models are models and any real people they see are really, really fabulous—socialites or movie stars. Since we're less about models and not at all about socialites or movie stars, we're more approachable—so we're often approached.

As I've noted, I am not a particularly pretty girl and certainly do not take a pretty picture. I know this, and it doesn't disturb me at all. I know I am prettier than my picture says I am, and I employ my strong denial tactics wherever I can. The best use of denial is my strategy for appearing on TV—which is to appear on TV, to say what I say and try to act normal, and then to never watch the tape. If a tree falls in the forest and nobody sees it, did it happen? If you look awful or, worse, stupid and graceless, why would you want to have that information? I just like to imagine that I was brilliant and leave it at that. Anyway, knowing that my career as any sort of model would be nasty, brutish, and short is a comfort to me, and I feel no need to be photographed extensively as a result.

But a great many women—no matter what they look like, no matter what their style—believe themselves to be gorgeous models underneath it all and that their pictures need to appear in top fashion magazines posthaste. I think the whole "oh, with all that makeup and all that retouching, Queen Elizabeth would look like Cindy Crawford!" wisdom has gotten to them, and they insist, insist that they would make fine models for *Lucky*. "What about little old me for one of those '*Lucky* Girl' pieces?" is a question I am asked every day by the most unlikely candidates. I sometimes think the whole self-esteem crisis is not quite the epidemic people are making it out to be.

It may be the more approachable style of *Lucky* that gets people in this mood. This was something so refreshing to hear about when we went out and got to meet *Lucky* readers in focus groups. Let me qualify all of this: You know I hate focus groups. I think they're the reason every perfume smells precisely like the last one and why New Coke happened and all the rest that's wrong with our troubled nation.

A focus group is the fifteen minutes of fame Andy Warhol promised us at last.

"Um, like, if I could just get a mascara that, um, doesn't clump??!!"

"Yeah! Like a mascara that doesn't clump!!"

The marketers are listening to you—*really* listening to you. They hang on your every word, perhaps even record or film it, and they take it seriously, they bring it back to their clients, and at last, you, tiny person, are heard: You want mascara that doesn't clump! It's like voting, but about something you have real opinions on. I hate focus groups.

Of course, if you're making the product they're commenting on, you can scorn the format all you like, but you listen. At *Elle*, we'd start by asking them if they like women's fashion magazines. Every single woman in the room would shake her head in disgust.

"No! I hate women's fashion magazines!"

"The models are too thin!"

"Nobody looks like that!"

"The clothes are too expensive!"

"They're ridiculous! I hate them, too!"

Well, what sorts of magazines do you subscribe to? was

always the next question. "Oh, *Vogue, Elle, W, Harper's Bazaar, Glamour . . .*"

At the *Lucky* focus groups, the conversation went a little differently. The focus group facilitator person would ask, "Who do you think this magazine is for?" and every woman in the room—the sixty-five-year-old and the seventeen-year-old alike—would reply, "It's aimed at people like me—me and my friends." They didn't even see us as a fashion magazine, despite the fact that we feature more fashion than most fashion magazines.

In much the way it probably feels to be summoned for and questioned in a focus group, I felt very important that I'd be asked to watch them. It was my second experience dealing with James Truman, after the terrible first-day, Beautyscene.com debacle. Authority figures make me nervous to begin with, and I found James Truman to be wildly handsome and brilliant, which made the whole thing a thousand times worse.

We were halfway through our first focus group in Chicago when he first appeared. Andrea (Linett, our creative director) and I had just gone through a laborious half-hour-long debate about whether to order Thai or Italian. We chose Thai and phoned in the order. James Truman (yes, I must use both names), too, took the decision very seriously and surveyed the two menu options carefully (what is it about what to order in while you're working?). "I think I'll have Thai," he said at last.

"That's so funny!" I said brightly. He and Andrea both looked at me (Andrea, because she already knew of my propensity to say idiotic things to James Truman, with a slight warning expression). "Because Andrea and I just ordered Italian, too!"

"No . . . Jean, um, we ordered Thai," Andrea said as gently as she could. She cleared her throat nervously. "James wants Thai, too. James, shall we add you to the order?"

The next time I saw him, I was yelling something over my shoulder as I came out of Kim's office. To the casual observer (say, the handsome James Truman), I probably sounded angry, but I wasn't. I was just being sarcastic. A bit later, I was on my way to lunch; I got into the elevator—and so did he. I felt he was too important a person to say hello to—doing so would have been overly familiar and presumptuous. So I looked up at the numbers of the floors, the way you're supposed to, with what I felt was an acceptable look of calm pleasantry. We finally reached the bottom; before the doors opened (interminable), he suddenly blurted, "Uh, are you all right?"

Panicked, I nodded. "It's just that I'm in a terrible hurry!" I said, looking at my watch for effect. I tore out of the elevator in what must have been the most inelegant exit in the history of Condé Nast. To make sure I was convincing, I ran all the way down Forty-third Street, just in case he was watching—and managed to stumble and break my heel. He was not, as it turned out, watching.

Things only got worse. The ultimate was an editorial meeting in Kim's office. Kim and James Truman were commenting on the annual barbeque at the CEO's house they'd attended the night before; fried chicken had been served.

"I had a party last night and we had fried chicken, too!" I felt compelled to offer.

"Well," said James Truman as he sat down beside me, "what will you be making for the Fourth of July?" (It was the next day.)

"Uh, um, I guess fried chicken again," I ventured lamely.

Everyone was silent; the topic had reached a dead and unspectacular end. For reasons unknown, I felt compelled to try to fix it; I continued on, as everyone stared in quiet horror.

"Uh, um, I don't actually *make* the fried chicken," I said. "I, uh, buy it at the store."

Authority I have my issues with, but authority and handsomeness are too much for me to deal with.

Perhaps it follows—or perhaps it doesn't—that I myself am a horrible boss. You'd think after ten or whatever years of it, I'd have sorted things out, but this is not the case. There are plenty of brilliant, talented operatives who've worked for me and still love me, but I think it is *because* they loved me (despite my many flaws) that they succeeded and because they loved me that I was able to govern somewhat reasonably.

Being the boss is trouble. Everyone and his brother has unworked-out authority issues that they project onto you with an enormous dollop of entitlement. "Hey, Mom! I dare you to yell at me and make me clean up my room!" That kind of thing. I had one woman, whom I'd done nothing but hire, and promote, and hire again, and promote again, quit over the phone on the day of the funeral of my much-loved grandmother. It's very easy to take it personally and think, Why me? Why do I deserve this? But there's no point.

The worst kind of boss, I've read, is me, the type who tries to be your friend. A nice buttoned-up, utterly dignified, and authoritative boss is the easiest to work for, because you know how to act, and you know you better not fuck up, so you do your best and you're happy at the end of the day. Instead, my sentences are full of un-PC, Ophelia-inflected I'm sorrys, which serve only to make everyone resentful.

I, meanwhile, resent their resentfulness. I want to point out the sorts of tyrants who run rampant in the magazine business, people who scream and yell and humiliate and fire like it's going out of style. That tack doesn't work, though, the "you don't know how good you have it": My husband does it all the time, pointing out how awful all the other husbands are. It makes me grit my teeth, glower, and curse under my breath rather than feel the rush of gratitude I think he's angling for.

I also can't fire people, which is a skill every boss needs to have. Because I was scarred by having to fire someone once (it wasn't a completely unjust firing, but it also wasn't a no-brainer and involved a vein popping out of the person's head as I thought I was speaking evenly and fairly about severance), I've enabled many others I should've fired to stay on and wreak havoc not only on my life, but on those of my talented and productive co-workers.

At *Lucky*, I even had a fellow editor come in and pretend she was firing me so I might get up the courage to do it myself (all the higher-ups were demanding I fire my lackluster assistant): "Jean, I think we both know this isn't what you want to be doing," she began. Thankfully, the assistant quit before I could get to her.

Lucky Style

The fashion closet at *Lucky* is a distinctly different place from the one at *Elle*. It's full of cool things that a real person might conceivably wear; at *Elle*, it was all fantasy, all the time. As a result, I really miss *Elle* on the nights I have black ties: There's no John Galliano fantasias or Versace extravaganzas to avail myself of.

One night, though, I pushed my luck anyway. They'll have something, I thought as I brought in an old, long black skirt and a pair of black strappy shoes that morning. "Anything?" I asked in the late afternoon. Umm, no, was the unequivocal answer.

I dug and I dug and, desperate, settled on an Urban Outfitters sweater that cost maybe $30. I went to the black tie, which was held in the superswank Cipriani building—movie stars everywhere, flowers, champagne. I slid into my seat. "Your top!" exclaimed the hostess, a vision in Oscar de la Renta. "I love it. Who made it?" Who asks that question? Who made it?

"Oh, it's vintage." I had to tell that lie about seventy times that night; never have I worn such a popular outfit. It just goes to show: Don't spend the money if you don't love it, because no one—not even the experts—knows the difference.

No, the thing I borrow most often from the *Lucky* fashion department is yoga ensembles. Though *Lucky* rarely does fitness stories, there's always something lackluster enough lying around that I can borrow when I forget to bring something for yoga. And, you know, it's a yoga class. No one cares what you're wearing.

My yoga class is not particularly glamorous, and the lights are often low. On occasion, however, the hip-hop mogul Russell Simmons appears in the class; I love him. It is not only the handsomeness of Russell Simmons, it is also the fact that he can do the splits frontways and then lie down on his stomach as if it were nothing. And he fights for an end to mandatory prison sentences and generally works to make the world a better place. Plus, when he was the It Guy and had just invented Phat Farm, and I was freelancing for *Seventeen*, he was one of the few celebrities who treated me nicely when I was assigned to interview him. So I see Russell Simmons from afar in class, worship silently, and move on.

One night there was nothing in the closet but a very large

pair of teal cotton shorts and a tight-fitting Pepto-Bismol-colored shirt. Naturally, I was late to class that day, and whom did I find myself right next to (in my yoga class, they pack us in so closely and work us so hard that by the end of class, you've probably exchanged more bodily fluids—primarily sweat—with the people next to you than if you'd slept with them several times in a grimy sleeping bag at a Burning Man festival), but Russell Simmons himself.

I attempted to rise above the ballooning teal shorts and focused, intently, on doing the best yoga I could. But because I was sweating so profusely—such was the effort I was making—and was wearing shorts rather than yoga pants, I found that in many of the poses I had become too slippery to manage anything and went crashing to the floor several times, landing in a billowy yet sodden pink-and-teal heap. Pretty.

I thought I might somehow redeem myself when I was invited to the Simmons home for the launch of Goddess, the new perfume by Kimora Lee Simmons (wife of Russell, quoted in *Vanity Fair* re: other women: "I will kick a bitch's ass").

"Yeah, we're in the same yoga class," I imagined saying coolly. In my carefully composed outfit, he'd never recognize me as the bumbling interloper of a few weeks before.

We were ferried out to the Simmons estate in New Jersey in enormous limousines. We hit traffic, and the limo lurched forward in a stomach-unsettling way. I felt particularly sorry for the three pregnant beauty editors in the car; we jounced along, forgoing the Cristal and chocolate-covered strawberries. When the gates at last opened, we were welcomed inside by a team of the most handsome men I have ever seen. But no Russell. The house itself was palatial; the scale, everywhere, was enormous. It was a little like in *The Nutcracker* when the tree grows and suddenly the presents around it tower over the players like skyscrapers. I passed a throw pillow the size of a VW Bug with the words *Om Shanti* inscribed on it.

Outside, there were fountains and huge topiaries galore. Dotted through the fountains and topiary were life-size statues of Greek god/goddess types. Also piles of caviar in great bowls. As I was searching the crowd for the always-glowing Mr. Simmons (to no avail), I kept detecting something—movement—out of the corner of my eye. To be sure, the crowd was mixing and milling about, but this movement was somehow different: It was the statues. The statues were actual life-size human beings, made up (the way makeup artist Joanne Gair famously full-body-makeup-ed Demi Moore for *Vanity Fair*) to resemble naked stone statues, fig leaves and all.

But no Russell. Kimora herself was gorgeous, friendly, vivacious, and, like her furniture, larger than life. Her extensions flowed past her behind, her laugh was loud, her voice authoritative, her body perfect.

I thoroughly enjoyed myself, despite my grave disappointment. We left, as always, with a bagful of goodies (perfume, etc.), this time including a face cookie emblazoned with the likeness of Kimora Lee. Face cakes and face cookies (where you give the bakery a picture of yourself and they somehow interpret it in icing) are hilarious things—at *Lucky*, we had several years where each person's birthday was marked with an ever more ridiculous face cake. Somehow, the picture of you never quite translates onto pastry the way you think it might.

Kimora's did not do her justice, not at all. I presented it to Adam, who got very excited. "This is genius!" he said, peering at it closely. He did not recognize Kimora Lee in the slightest; the icing had stretched her face into unrecognizable contortions, eyes over here, mouth over there, cleavage out to here.... "A prostitute energy bar!" he exclaimed, turning it in his hand. "You're a prostitute, you're too busy, so you just pop one of these and keep going!"

The face-cake/cookie artists do the opposite magic when presented with the image of a *Lucky* staffer to interpret in icing; getting one of *our* face cakes is a little like having your picture taken with one of those sun-damage cameras, where you see, in unflinching detail, what you're going to look like when you're seventy-five. Given the choice, I'd prefer the prostitute energy-bar style to the *Mrs. Doubtfire* thing my face-cake had going on.

Along with the face cake hegemony, *Lucky* staffers often show up in the same clothes. Unlike anywhere else in America, at *Lucky* aping someone else's style is not only permissible, it is celebrated. If two people arrive at work wearing the same outfit, Polaroids are taken immediately and the pictures are tacked onto a great wall reserved specifically for such style conflagrations. If someone arrives in a fabulous new item, she's asked, over and over, "Where'd you get that?" and we all immediately flock to the store and buy one apiece. It's opposite the way things usually go—two socialites appearing at the same gala in the same ball gown, disaster. Two celebs caught wearing the same outfit, ever—the actual wearing can occur weeks apart, but the paparazzi magazines will pair the two pictures on a page anyway—awful. At *Lucky*, a clothing item is closer to a great mascara or a cute new lip gloss shade: You share it with your friends.

The editors and their widely varying sense(s) of style are often featured in the magazine—me among them. While I like to think of myself as daring and avante-garde, whenever my style is featured, to my great chagrin, I get sensible-classic-Ann-Taylor girl, rather than the groundbreaking downtowner/bohemian mold I imagine myself fitting. It's another sort of mirror, one I'm not as far along in coming to terms with. "It's not that you're so classic," Andrea will say, backpedaling furiously. "It's just, you know, we need a contrast for this story, so you wear the crewneck sweater, okay?" I know, in my heart of hearts, that she's only reporting the truth, but still, I can't accept it.

The truth can be hard. When I get tired and I want to see someone truly blanch, I try out my style on the *Lucky* fashion department. Certain items capture my imagination, and, like a child with a favorite toy, I wear them to death—past death, even.

I had a big beauty event to go to, and I'd worked out the dress and the shoes. They were the perfect shoes: champagne panne-velvet kitten-heel sandals, old in a "New Orleans debutante emerges as the most significant artist of her time" sort of way. I trotted it all out before the fashion department, imagining the moment when they all gasped and demanded to know where I got the shoes. I would shrug and say, "Old Louboutin," in an offhand and glamorous way.

They looked me up and down; all eyes, as I'd secretly predicted, stopped at my feet.

"Oh no," said one.

"You're not serious."

"Um . . . you need to throw those out now."

"Jean, they have mold on them!" The truth is hard. So I've had to replace them. Except there's no replacing with shoes, is there?

I wish I could say I run around correcting the makeup faux

pas of my bumbling co-workers, but it's just not so. They've all got it pretty well figured out. Though Kim does demand I apply her concealer if she's forgotten to book a makeup artist for some appearance or another; people always assume that a beauty editor would be better at putting on makeup or deciding on a hairstyle than your average stylish person, and I have to say, I fall down in this category completely. I can dab on concealer, yes, but tell you whether you need blue or green eyeliner? I'm no makeup artist. That's why I interview them when I'm writing my articles rather than simply making pronouncements.

Even when we aren't sharing our style sources, our shopping instincts are shockingly similar. The best example of this phenomenon was when we all went to Los Angeles for the *Lucky* launch party there. As with all parties, the torture part was what to wear; Sofia Coppola was involved, so we were a thousand times more tortured, as she epitomizes all that is stylish in our world today. James Truman would also be in attendance, sending me over the edge. Once in Los Angeles, we all shopped furiously, the impending glamour like dark clouds gathering. We drove here, we drove there: Melrose, Robertson, Rodeo. There were jeans, there were T-shirts, there were necklaces, but there was nothing to wear to the party. The day of the party, after a meeting in the morning, we all retired to our respective rooms at the hotel, to call the office, e-mail something . . . I, of course, still desperate for something to wear, went back to my room and immediately called a cab.

"Take me to Fred Segal," I said.

As I emerged from the cab in the parking lot of Fred Segal, two other cab doors were opening simultaneously. Funny, I thought, people in Los Angeles never take cabs. Out stepped a silver-spray-painted Birkenstock—couldn't be anyone but

Andrea Linett. Out of the other, the fashion news director. We looked at one another sheepishly. So much for phoning the office.

Once inside, whom should we bump into but the art director? And suddenly there was Kim, looking just as sheepish. There was nothing to do but laugh and start shopping. We passed the café; inside was Leilani, our cover model, picking at a salad. A *Lucky* girl is a *Lucky* girl.

Eerily, we also spotted Coppola herself, chatting on her cell phone, clearly not worrying about what to wear that night. The afternoon wore on; the party loomed. Frantic, with the help of all my co-workers I settled on a short-sleeved (though I hate my arms) purple-sequined T-shirt from a designer I loathe. The shirt was somehow fabulous, so much so that I grew concerned that hipster partygoers would ask me where I got it, forcing me to reveal the awful truth, the desperately unchic designer. Should such a situation arise, I decided, once again I'd have to fall back on the "vintage" defense.

Hair and makeup had to fall a little by the wayside, since we'd spent so much time deciding what to wear. But I found a Delux lip gloss that matched the purple in the shirt, put on a little eyeliner, and made it happen.

The party was so full of attractive, happening L.A. operatives that I had to have a drink or two. I roamed from room to room, trying to look purposeful, at home. When things got rough (I really am no good at parties, as you may have observed by now; I didn't yet know anyone at *Lucky* well enough to engage in a fake conversation), I went to the bathroom and applied the fabulous lip gloss. No one asked me about the shirt.

At last I ran into a demiceleb I loathe. She was wearing the most hideous dress I've ever seen. "Omigod, I love your dress!"

I exclaimed. Very Fashionista of me. Giving my gender a bad name and all.

"Do you? It's ———," she said, beaming proudly. Naturally, it was the same designer. "I *love* your shirt."

"Vintage," I said, and I never wore it again.

I did haul it back home with me, and several months later it reappeared, in a dress-up game going on between my eight-year-old daughter and her friend Ana. India was naturally not the one wearing the sparkly shirt, given her staunch ungirliness in all things. Her complete oblivion re: glamour (my lipsticks, in her hands, becoming an army of slugs, for example) always reminds me—stunningly so—of my mother.

But there they were upstairs in my room with Adam, India looking like a miniature escapee from the Castro with an enormous policeman hat balanced on her head, Ana glittering in the purple-pailletted shirt. Gradually the game shifted; the costumes went by the wayside, and they sidled up to my basket full of makeup, in front of the mirror.

They went for mascara and lipstick, primarily, with a little eyeliner (Adam and I were of course called in for the actual application). A huge amount of laughing and irritated eye blinking and quizzical lip pursing ensued, and then they turned toward the mirror.

Ana, the way you or I might, turned, cocked her head, looked herself in the eye, gave a small secret smile . . . mirror face, as previously described. I've got one, and so do you.

India, on the other hand, in much the way either of her grandparents might if presented with the same situation, burst into peals of laughter. Raucous, blurted laughter, as if she were looking into a funhouse mirror and were delighted at the extreme ridiculousness of the distortions it reflected back. As if she'd just been in a food fight, or rolled in the mud, and couldn't believe how silly she looked. Although it's true that an eight-year-old does look faintly silly with mascara on, the reaction far outstripped the reality.

When they finally map the human genome, they're going to find a glamour gene, and there's going to be something about skipping generations in there. Perhaps my daughter will be the one to discover it, there swimming among the enzymes and coenzymes and ATP and ribozymes.

When she goes to accept the Nobel Prize for it, her ancient, foundation-caked mother will try to get her to put on a little gloss, maybe the subtlest bit of perfume, before she ascends to the dias. It's going to be rough.

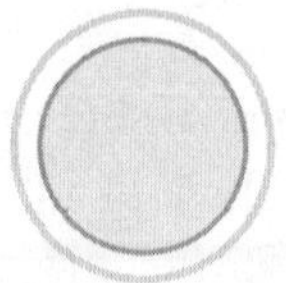

About the Author

Jean Godfrey-June is the beauty editor of *Lucky* magazine. She lives in New York with her husband and two children.